M000210475

ANOTHER DAY IN THE MONKEY'S BRAIN

ANOTHER DAY
in the
MONKEY'S
BRAIN

RALPH MITCHELL SIEGEL

Center for Molecular and Behavioral Neuroscience

Rutgers University

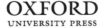

OXFORD
UNIVERSITY PRESS

OXFORD
UNIVERSITY PRESS

Oxford University Press, Inc., publishes works that further
Oxford University's objective of excellence
in research, scholarship, and education.

Oxford   New York
Auckland   Cape Town   Dar es Salaam   Hong Kong   Karachi
Kuala Lumpur   Madrid   Melbourne   Mexico City   Nairobi
New Delhi   Shanghai   Taipei   Toronto

With offices in
Argentina   Austria   Brazil   Chile   Czech Republic   France   Greece
Guatemala   Hungary   Italy   Japan   Poland   Portugal   Singapore
South Korea   Switzerland   Thailand   Turkey   Ukraine   Vietnam

Copyright © 2012 by Oxford University Press, Inc.
Introduction Copyright © 2012 by Oliver Sacks

Published by Oxford University Press, Inc.
198 Madison Avenue, New York, New York 10016
www.oup.com

Oxford is a registered trademark of Oxford University Press

All rights reserved. No part of this publication may be reproduced,
stored in a retrieval system, or transmitted, in any form or by any means,
electronic, mechanical, photocopying, recording, or otherwise,
without the prior permission of Oxford University Press.

Library of Congress Cataloging-in-Publication Data
Siegel, Ralph Mitchell, 1958-2011.
Another day in the monkey's brain/Ralph Mitchell Siegel.
p. cm.
Includes bibliographical references and index.
ISBN 978-0-19-973434-4 (hardback: alk. paper) 1. Siegel, Ralph Mitchell,
1958-2011. 2. Neurophysiologists—United States—Biography. I. Title.
RC339.52.S553A3 2012
616.80092—dc23
[B]
2011046543

1 3 5 7 9 8 6 4 2
Printed in USA on acid-free paper

To my truest love, my wife, Jasmine: holding hands in a yellow wood, we took the road less travelled by; this has made all the difference in our journey.

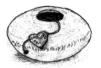

"Sweet-in-the-bowl"

To my children, my Dashiel and my Zoe, my endless source of "happy thoughts." I soar, with hopes and dreams for you, for your literary and scientific selves. You taught me the art of making toe soup, and your encouragement and query echo eternally.

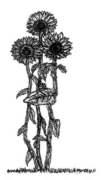

"We all stand upon the shoulders of giants."

And to my cherished family and friends, my valued colleagues and community members: your relational roles to me often intersect, but I am confident that each one of you will know how you have contributed your inspiration, encouragement, and willingness to be a part of my greater family, and feel the depth of my gratitude for your boundless generosity in spirit, in time, and in energy.

The Question

To ask the hard question is simple;
Asking at meeting
With the simple glance of acquaintance
To what these go
And how these do:
To ask the hard question is simple,
The simple act of the confused will.
But the answer
Is hard and hard to remember . . .

—W. H. Auden

CONTENTS

by Oliver Sacks

I first met Ralph Siegel in 1973. He was just a teenager then, and his uncle, a dean at the Albert Einstein College of Medicine, introduced us. Ralph, at fifteen, was passionate about science and already pondering the relation of brain to mind— "the hard question" that was always the center of his thought.

"He's very bright," I said to his uncle. "Extremely bright. He's too bright to be a doctor; he should be a physiologist." Twenty years later, when Ralph was a physiologist, but had no tenure as yet and was earning only the miserable salary that post-docs get, his father looked at me reproachfully and said, only half-joking, "You prevented my son earning a decent living! If he was a doctor, he would have a house in the suburbs and a decent income, and not be living hand-to-mouth as he does now."

Ralph and I re-met, met properly, at a concert in 1987. We were both sitting in the top circle (in England they say "with the gods") at Carnegie Hall, and Ralph chanced to be sitting a few rows behind me. We had seen each other, extremely briefly, the previous year when I had visited the Salk Institute—Ralph was closely attached to Francis Crick then; he was, to some degree, as Crick put it, one of Crick's many "sons-in-science." When Ralph saw that I had a notebook on my lap and was writing nonstop throughout the concert, he knew the bulky figure ahead of him had to be me. He came up and introduced himself at the end of the concert (I was writing all through the interval), and I recognized him at once—not by his face (most faces look the same to me), but by his flaming red hair.

I suggested supper together at the Carnegie Deli, thinking he would relish one of their famous meat sandwiches—each contained almost a pound of meat. But Ralph was appalled by the idea of pastrami: he was a vegetarian then, and he could not bear the idea of eating anything with neurons. So he had a salad, and I followed suit. Ralph was curious—what had I been writing about through the entire concert? He asked whether I was wholly unconscious of the music. (The program included Mozart's great G-minor Mass and, after the interval, his Requiem.) No, I said, I was conscious of the music all the time, and not just as background. I said that Nietzsche used to write at concerts, too; he especially loved Bizet, and would say, "Bizet makes me a better philosopher."

I said I felt that Mozart made me a better neurologist, and that I had been writing about a patient I had seen who had become suddenly unable to see or imagine color following a road accident (and possibly a slight stroke in addition). Ralph was excited; he had heard of this patient, for I had described him to Crick earlier in the year. Ralph's own work was exploring the visual system (using monkeys) in Torsten Wiesel's lab at Rockefeller University, but he would love, he said, to explore more with the colorblind painter, who could tell him exactly what he was seeing (or not seeing). He outlined half a dozen simple but crucial tests that could help pinpoint at what stage the construction of color had broken down in the painter's brain.

I had never heard the word "construction" used in this way before, and I began to realize, in that first meal together, that Ralph immediately thought in deep physiological terms, while neurologists, myself included, often contented ourselves with the surface features, the phenomenology of brain disease or damage, with little thought of the precise mechanism involved . . . and no thought at all of the ultimate question of how experience and consciousness emerged from brain activity. In that first meeting with Ralph, I realized how far neuroscience had come since my own physiology days in the early 1950s, and how, for Ralph, all the questions he explored in the monkey brain, the insights he so patiently collected one by one, were always pointing to that ultimate question. I said I would check with Mr. I., the painter, but I was sure he would welcome Ralph and any insight he could bring to the situation (as he had welcomed Bob Wasserman, an ophthalmologist friend of mine).

So it was in Ralph that I confronted, and felt confronted with, a very acute neuroscientific mind and realized that the two of us, with our different orientations, could complement each other, form a team, and do work which neither of us could do alone.

In that first dinner at the Carnegie Deli, a friendship began, as well as a partnership, which has lasted ever since. We were both keen cyclists and took long rides together. When, by coincidence, we were both invited to Australia, Ralph not only helped me prepare an inaugural lecture for the newly founded Centre for the Mind, but also came snorkeling and scuba diving with me and my family on the Great Barrier Reef. (My brother was very taken with Ralph, and called him "Dr. Stentor" because of his loud voice, a voice that sometimes enabled him to dispense with a microphone when he lectured or presented papers at scientific meetings.)

Ralph, who had been indifferent to things religious before (he was a Jewish atheist, as I am) was converted into a much more active and deeply felt Judaism after spending a Friday evening, an Erev Shabbat, with my brother and his family in Sydney. (This was ironic, because my brother himself, though fond of the old rituals and prayers, was not particularly observant or much of a believer. Freeman Dyson once wrote, "I am a practicing Christian, but not a believing one," and my brother felt much the same way about being a Jew.) After his Australian visit, Ralph's life took on a religious dimension, and he became an observant Jew (and, as far as I could judge, a believing one).

Ralph's wife, Jasmine, also has a background in experimental neuroscience, and when they returned from Ralph's sabbatical year in San Diego, she began working in Ralph's lab at Rutgers, training monkeys and generally helping to organize and carry out the experiments that Ralph designed. They have long been partners in work, as well as husband and wife and parents. Although some people are horrified by the idea of animal research and the idea of monkeys with electrodes in their brains, "forced" to do various tasks and tests while their brain activity is monitored, Ralph and Jasmine both are animal lovers, and are particularly concerned with the monkeys in their charge. When I had an old black-and-white TV set, Ralph asked if he could have it for his monkeys, so they would not get bored.

Ralph came with me to see the colorblind painter many times. Together with Bob Wasserman and Semir Zeki, we published a poster presentation at the annual Society for Neuroscience meeting in 1988. Ralph also became close with a friend of mine who has Tourette's Syndrome. With his colleague Howard Poizner at Rutgers, he did some fascinating experiments which showed that Tourette's, while sometimes a heavy burden to bear, can allow people to make movements and reach out for targets far more quickly than normal; this demonstration of "superspeed" in a

"Touretter" attracted much attention when presented as a poster at another Neuroscience meeting.

There is a chapter in this book, "Triumvirate," about Ralph's close collaboration and friendship with two remarkable young research scientists. But there was also another sort of triumvirate, that of Ralph with two physicians, Bob Wasserman and myself. We first came together in the case of the colorblind painter; we came together again in the case of "Virgil," a blind man whose vision was restored at the age of fifty (he found it almost impossible to accommodate to this, to changing his mode of life and identity, after a lifetime of being blind). Our third visual collaboration was with "Stereo Sue," a gifted stereoblind woman who gained stereo vision in middle age and not only accommodated to the new visual gift, but also delighted in it, finding her life much enriched. The case of Stereo Sue led to our writing a letter together for *Science* about the unexpected potentials for regaining at least a partial but very useful degree of vision, even in those virtually blind from birth.

Ralph is a good natural mathematician, with a degree in physics, and finds computational neuroscience—making models or simulations of neurological systems—much to his liking. He was intrigued when I told him about the complex and beautiful recurrent geometrical patterns one might hallucinate in a visual migraine aura, and he was able to simulate its basic patterns on a neural network. In 1992 we included this work in an appendix to my book on *Migraine*. Ralph's mathematical and physical intuition led him to feel that chaos might also be central to natural processes of all kinds, and to every sort of science, from quantum mechanics to neuroscience. This led in 1990 to another collaboration between us, an appendix called "Chaos and Awakenings" in my book *Awakenings*.

Ralph has loved his time at the Salk Institute and the friend-ships he made there before moving East, and each summer goes back to the Salk—summers for him and his family are spent in La Jolla, where he can watch the windsurfers and hang gliders, go for long walks, cycle, and renew or form lasting bonds. A decade ago, I began joining him for short periods there every couple of years and started to feel myself part of this wonder-fully varied and original community.

It is rare to be at once a neurophysiological researcher, a theoretical neuroscientist, and a computational neuroscientist drawn to synthetic neural modeling, but Ralph is all three, inseparably. These passions for science, and the insatiable yet patient curiosity which makes doing science so hard, so time-consuming, but at the same time so joyful, have been central in Ralph's emotional life no less than his intellectual one. The physiologist Vernon Mountcastle has been one of the great influences in Ralph's life (as in the lives of hundreds of other young scientists). Mountcastle found it hard to retire from lab-oratory work at age seventy (though over ninety now, he is still incessantly active, writing books, distilling the wisdom of a very long and wonderfully productive lifetime). Soon after he retired from his lab, Vernon Mountcastle wrote me a most moving letter, including these words:

I am still actively engaged in scholarly activity, but I miss laboratory work in a way that is difficult to describe. It has always been my heart's joy, and my own experience has always been that even the most trivial original discovery of one's own evokes a special kind of ecstasy—it is almost like falling in love for the first time, all over again!

This, too, is how it has been for Ralph, and it is this passion, along with the frustrations and sometimes torments of a life in science, blended superbly with the personal, which is so clearly and movingly conveyed in *Another Day in the Monkey's Brain*.

Doing science is so often presented as a logical sequence of fortunate events. This is not so often the truth.

Serendipity plays its role, as in the story of the discovery of orientation tuning by David Hubel and Torsten Wiesel in 1961. Twenty years later, in front of a standing-room-only audience attending the annual Society for Neuroscience meeting at the Church of the Open Door in Los Angeles, Hubel told the story of how they had not been able to activate any neurons in the striate cortex, the second step of the visual system, with any of their standard visual stimuli of circles and spots. Then one day, as they inserted in frustration yet another slide with a small circular cutout at its center, the neuron went crazy, sputtering and crackling. It turned out that the slide insertion presented a sharp, straight edge at just the correct orientation to excite the neuron. Chance favored their prepared minds, the modern study of vision was launched, and twenty years later, in 1981, they became Nobel laureates.

Dreams, too, are often vital in the doing of science. Think of Kékule's dream of a whirling snake chasing its tail in a circle and his subsequent discovery of the benzene ring. Otto Loewi had to twice dream the experiments demonstrating chemical transmission; in these experiments, he discovered the first neurotransmitter, *Vagusstoff*, now called acetylcholine.

Still, the descriptions of doing science are often written by people whose views of past, present, and future paint an orderly progression, a high-minded undertaking toward the greater good.

For me (and many of my friends), science is intricately woven into our daily lives. We inwardly seek to resolve our drive to succeed, to understand the impenetrable scientific problems, while also loving our families and the meaning of our personal lives. Our intellectual powers do not necessarily prepare us to strike a balance between the two.

This book is the story of part of my life in science, and, at least for me, in the beginning, there was little separation between the science and myself. As must be, my passage through time engendered a journey through space, a spiritual journey. In these pages, I describe events of science, events of growing. Each day, each step affected both my understanding of the brain and mind, and my understanding of self.

————

I began my studies of brain and mind, oddly enough, because I had little understanding of my identity and place in the world. At the end of 1976, our country's bicentennial year, I thought that answers to my personal adolescent anguish lay in academics—in Freudian psychology, in Aristotle's *De Anima*, and in the studies of nerve fibers in a dish. Three disparate choices lay in front of me: Philosophy, Psychology, and Physiology—the historical pillars of the study of mind and (once it was known to matter) brain.

Nature and nurture conspired with my natural bent toward the scientific approach, and I decided to follow in the footsteps of my father—a biologist and a dentist—toward a stream whose torrent had been loosened by Hubel and Wiesel. All I needed to do was to step in and let the current carry me.

As an undergraduate, I read others' reasons for their choices. Eric Kandel's preface to the *Cellular Basis of Behavior*[1] promised a revolution in the science of brain: "Until this [experimental] work in invertebrates, the distance between the study of the physiological mechanisms of behavior and traditional psychology was often considered the widest between any related scientific disciplines." Right or wrong, I read the phrase "traditional psychology" to refer to that of Sigmund Freud, Carl Jung, and R. D. Laing. I thought Kandel was saying we could have a science revealing the great complexity of mind based on understanding a shell-less gastropod, *Aplysia*.

This expectation that the understanding of *Aplysia's* simple circuits would presage that of higher cognition was echoed by

Stephen Kuffler and John G. Nicholls.[2] "As physiologists ...
we are convinced that behind each problem that appears extraordinarily complex and insoluble there lies a simplifying principle
that will lead to an unraveling of the events."

So I apprenticed to become a physiologist, to learn the fine
details of neurons and synapses, of *Vagusstoff.*

I was also fortunate to find a psychologist who helped me
open some doors of my own consciousness. And so a dichotomy
began in my search for who I was. I learned about "me" through
a journey of self-exploration, and I learned about the brain at
its most elementary details of channel, membrane, and synapse.
For many years, the two studies—physiology and self—were
separate, and the big question lay dormant: How could channels, membranes, and synapses give rise to perception, thought,
and, ultimately, to consciousness?

In the chapters that follow, I bring these two strands together.

There is still no answer to the hard question of the origins
of consciousness. Although consciousness is built from—and
of—the physical, the biological, and the chemical, consciousness's complexity will always exhibit, expound, exemplify,
explode, and emerge in the most illogical and unexpected forms
of behavior.

ONE

A DAY IN THE MONKEY'S BRAIN

It is once again my first day back at The Salk Institute, my intellectual home. I do science that represents the best of a comingled and open community. Each day I continue my journey to understanding the nature of consciousness, not at the phenomenological level, as a philosopher of mind might, but as an experimentalist.

I tire easily of long discourses—"distractions," as my good friend Tom Albright would say. I never drank deeply of Hume or Kant, never cared about materialism or the nature of reason. Dualism concerned me, as I could see the mind and brain only as one indistinguishable whole. What mind is, brain is. It was not a matter of levels of description. Destroying the brain destroyed the mind. Tearing out a small part of the brain, as a stroke might, took away a mechanistic atom of a person.[1]

So far, my journey toward understanding the nature of consciousness has been slow, taking many forms and leading me on many side trips to uncharted lands. These adventures distract, yet they are the foundational support for the much more difficult experimental questions. Each problem is almost a toy problem, an experiment in knowing how to proceed.

The questions address visual perception. Each of us has a clear visual picture of the world in front of us. This picture, this stuff we call reality, is wholly a construction of neuronal process. There is no movie screen in our head and there is no one to watch it. How is this visual representation formed in our head?

Since 1958, the year of my birth, tremendous strides in delimiting the first steps of this visual representation have been made by a mechanistic dissection of the neural elements. This dissection has revealed the following: light passes through the lens of the eye, a simple camera-like apparatus that provides an inverted image. Particular cells, honed by evolution, efficiently and sensitively transform the light energy into graded electrical signals at the rear of the eyeball—the retina. The particular mathematical transforms of the electrical signals are well, if not completely, understood.[2] An image arriving in the eye is elegantly modified to yield maximal information and essential characteristics.[3]

These early steps of understanding neuronal processing have succeeded through slow and meticulous collaboration by the experimentalist and the computational theorist. There is the hope, stated again and again, that these principles embodied in the early sensory system, principles gained through great tenacity, will apply to the stuff some of us really want to know about. We hope to answer Wilder Penfield's challenge, engraved on the retina of every McGill undergraduate who walks up University Avenue past the Montreal Neurological Institute: "The problem of neurology is to understand man himself."

There is little that scientists agree on to explain even visual perception, let alone consciousness. There is still no complete answer to the question of consciousness. My experiments in finding the truth are bound tightly to the doing of science. In my process, experiments to ask these hard questions are not objective and crystalline events. I cannot, in the concrete towers of the Salk staring out at the blue ocean, just plan a study. I wander both metaphorically and physically through ideas; I barge in on young and old colleagues. I hear a seminar, triggering unrelated memories of a lecture heard in graduate school. There is a convergence of the old and new in my head, a sense of delight, of illumination, an asking of a question that sometimes falls on deaf ears or that at other times evolves into a heated exchange. The ground is littered with the refuse of our doing of brain science. Sometimes a beautiful idea is orphaned, left mewing.

A small crowd of scientists races down the road to pick up the fruits of a chance discovery, a seemingly crucial piece of data, a new tool. I can see those left behind incessantly following their own ideas, dinosaurs in a time of small, agile mammals. And rarely do I see a scientist willfully step off the path, knowing a contribution is complete, content to leave the journey to the rest of us.

Each of us on this road is a collector. There are giants, as Newton said, upon whose shoulders we stand. But at this early stage, no one knows whose shoulders to stand on, how the journey will end, or even whether we will recognize the journey's end when we get to it.

Each day I place an electrode, a photon, a mathematical formula, a paper, a theory into the monkey's brain. Each day I hope for illumination. Each day I fail, and each day my experiments are infinitesimally closer to truth.

TWO

A Short Salk Story

As I walked past the East Buildings, I raised my eyes to the horizon. And perched on top of the March of Dimes steps was Bob Lizarraga. Now, Bob has been here at the Salk forever. He tells '60s-era stories of massive parties in unfinished research spaces, torrid romances in miniature elevators expressly designed to go up to the ivory tower studies. He also tells true stories, such as that of the first day the board of the March of Dimes, the primary fundraiser, came to view the finished product. Though the travertine marble had been laid and the Greek proportioned steps to the great courtyard were done, the words paying tribute to the March of Dimes were not yet completed. It was late in the evening when Bob discovered this.

The following words were to be engraved on the risers of the steps, beginning at eye level as you approached the Salk from the east and dropping below successively as you ascended to the entrance: "The National Foundation—March of Dimes—Led by Basil O'Connor—Established the Salk Institute—1960."

In a true burst of 1960s, youthful, can-do energy, so typifying the start of the Kennedy years, Bob and his friends found some two-by-four pieces of lumber, painted them to match the travertine marble, and carefully stenciled in gold the necessary words.

They worked through the night, and when the painting was done, propped the lumber in place at the front of the riser of each stair, and so the Salk was opened to its funders, who were none the wiser about what had transpired. The way Bob told it, no one even knew that the stairs had been left undone. What inspired that small crew, most of them no more than twenty years old, to stay up through the night to put the finishing touches on a new research building?

Today as I approached, Bob was talking to the construction supervisor and holding his hard hat in hand. It was the first time I had seen him since returning to the Salk. I thought of some quips like "Who needs a hard hat with a head as hard as yours," but his smile and outstretched hand deflated the New Yorker in me. He welcomed me back by saying, "I see the security guards ignored my instructions." In I had come.

I told him what a pleasure it was to have arrived for the summer. Bob said, "There was this Harvard professor used to come back every summer. He used those air tables with the copper cages around them. We made everything for him. He won the Nobel Prize."

I laughed as we both gazed out to the Pacific horizon, our feet slowly stepping across Jonas Salk's words embedded in the marble below our feet:

> Hope lies in dreams, in imagination
> and in the courage of those who
> dare to make dreams into reality.
>
> Jonas Salk

Bob went on to tell me how they used to make all sorts of scientific equipment for this Harvard guy. "At first there was no air table, so we would build a box of steel and fill it with sand to damp out the vibrations. And the machine shop would make him these little devices for moving electrodes around."

"Micromanipulators?"

"Yes, that's right. The machine shop could make anything in those days. He would come in every summer and tell you about another new idea he had."

I thought to myself. Who could this be? He shouldn't be hard to identify. Harvard professor, summers at Salk, microelectrodes, Nobel Prize? It sounded like an early neuroscientist. It would take two minutes on Google.

And Bob said, "Koo.., Koofer."

And I said, "Kuffler."

"That's right."

Stephen Kuffler never got the Nobel Prize. He died too soon, in 1980, but his prodigal sons David Hubel and Torsten Wiesel, who had first worked together in Kuffler's lab, received the prize the following year. They all shared it, even if one died a bit soon. Kuffler was renowned for selecting the ideal research preparation to match the research question. He was a founder of our field, a founder of the first department of neurobiology at Harvard. His mentors were Bernard Katz and John Eccles, connecting back to the very origins of modern-day neuroscience.

Twenty years ago, when I first met Bob, he was a draftsman for the Salk. I did not know of his late-night antics. And as we knew each other better, I found him to be a complex man. I was surprised when his wedding took place down at the westernmost reach of the Institute, at sunset, with the waterfall as a counterpoint to the musicians. (I would never have gotten married at my research institute in Newark.) He would give haircuts in a fenced-in crib in one of the interstitial spaces lined with magazine pages of unusually coiffed women. It was in his barber's chair that I heard stories of him working with Nobel laureates and other scientists to create their institute and keep it going.

What is an Institute? Does it exist outside the realm of physicality? Jonas Salk started with a simple idea, and the idea gained substance, funding, cement, rebar, travertine marble, and an architectural vision. Time passed and the Institute foundered financially. But many wealthy people continued to buy into Salk's dream. And it has endured well. Walking about its buildings, you can see the gold letters of Aristotle S. Onassis

Laboratory on the glass walls in the lower level of North Building. The William B. Hearst Research Center's brass plaque of 1976 lies at the Court level of the South Wing.

Salk's ideal has continued to be articulated and defined by the scientists drawn here. I have always believed that the Institute is run by hard-nosed, aggressive, extremely competitive, and brilliant scientists who nonetheless share a dream. The contrast is hard to fathom. Many of the senior people here could command either a research center of their own elsewhere or a successful startup, yet they stay and keep the Salk going.

There is a march, a progression of keepers of the Salk. Frederic de Hoffmann saved the Institute from Jonas Salk's financial mishandling, bringing to bear his expertise from General Atomics. Working with Max Cowan, Freddie placed the focus on science, while the other element of Jonas's dream— the element of humanism—went into hibernation, awaiting another time. After Freddie died, Renato Dulbecco stepped into the leadership breach. The next keeper in the succession was Francis Crick—at great cost to Francis's health. One year, I recall walking with Francis in the rain at the annual Society for Neuroscience meeting and asking what he was doing. His chest was scarred with the remnants of heart surgery. He said, "It is my turn to give *the Institute* back something after all it gave me."

"The Institute." A living entity that dreams. Not the scientists who dare to dream, not Jonas Salk's dream of a cross-cultural artistic and scientific haven, but the Salk Institute's dream, which is daily not only dared but also demands to be made into reality.

THREE

My First Encounter with Francis Crick

I first found Francis Crick while interviewing for a postdoctoral position at the Salk Institute. I knew he was there, and I knew he was my father's scientific hero, who had at once both removed the mystery from the question "What is life?"—so well posed by Schrödinger—and injected all the excitement back into biology. With my closest friend, Ehud Isacoff, I rehearsed for my presentation to Crick and made jokes about what I would say. None of this was real. What was real was that at two o'clock in the afternoon, I walked across Salk's courtyard to my first real ivory tower.

I was wearing new bright green running sneakers. They were my best shoes in 1983. My shirt was pressed, and all I carried was my hopes. The sneakers crossed over the river that lies pointing to the equinox. I headed up into the tower. As I came through the door there was a long corridor, completely in teak. At the end of the hallway was a desk. I started down the hallway. My fluorescent sneakers squeaked with every step on the polished wood floor. I walked fifty feet. I was self-conscious. Francis's secretary, Betty, announced me, and I went into his office. Francis's desk was angled slightly so he could look out his windows. His windows were at the west end of the Institute. Next to it, facing in the same direction, was a chair. I sat down. I looked out at the view. I looked to my left at this massive head, this spectacular view. Three windows of the Pacific Ocean, with nothing in the distance except California scrub and hang gliders.

I cannot remember just what happened, but in no time I was rattling on about my research. We know that neurons talk to each other across tiny gaps called synapses. The postsynaptic treelike structure of the dendrites modulated the effect of the neurotransmitter released from boutons; this had been extensively studied. I spoke of the presynaptic modulation of transmitter release as if it could change our entire notion of how neurons conversed.

I now know that my doctoral thesis used an outdated method to indirectly examine an expired experimental question. But Francis's attentions led me to exalted heights. Perhaps I did babble or maybe I spoke truths. But Francis listened and asked me harder questions about my work than anyone had before. It seemed he absorbed the entire issue instantly and placed it into an internal schema lodged in his massive temporal lobes, from which emerged just the right questions.

This was the first time I had seen anyone do this. Francis's memory was prodigious and he thought with great speed. Many times in seminars during the twenty years following that meeting, I watched him look almost asleep, his head weighted on one hand, eyes closed. At the end, he would ask that one question the speaker was not ready for, the question that illuminated the problem.

After a while Francis said it was time for tea. He pointed out that he would have coffee. I liked my tea black, and Betty brought a tray in with everything on it. It was dignified and simple. She also brought some almond cookies. They were hard with a single sliver in the middle. One cookie per plate. I reached over and lifted the cookie with my thumb and fingertip and pressed to crack the cookie in half. It was hard. It broke. Half went on the teak floor skittering quite a distance away, crumbs scattering everywhere. And Francis kept looking out at the hang gliders we could see in the distance, watching them glide and loop and spin in the afternoon sun, peaceful. It was an auspicious beginning.

Make no mistake; the hard work of science is in answering questions, but formulating the questions can be the difference between success and new knowledge, or failure and years spent traveling toward a dead end.

FOUR

CHAOS THROUGH THE LOOKING GLASS

The prevailing view of cortex is that of a machine. Each cortical area performs some operation and then passes on the result. An integral part of this model is that the system itself does not vary. However, both thought and cortical processing are flexible. This flexibility is due to the fantastic complexity inherent in large numbers. There are billions and billions of neurons and uncountable synaptic connections. Each neuron is a highly complex computing device. From the almost unknowable *number* of possibilities arises our species' individuality and genius.

Still, it is hard to imagine how the complexity of thought arises in a fixed type of computing machine. The world is variable, and so are we. Gerald Edelman put it succinctly: "The world is not like a piece of tape with a fixed sequence of symbols for the brain to read."[1]

Let's consider more closely a hard problem to solve. At first glance, it looks as though it ought to be cracked by a computer, yet it turned to be much, much harder. In 1967, the pre-Power-Point age, Leon Glass, a biological theorist, discovered by chance a set of unexpected visual stimuli while photocopying overhead transparencies of his lecture notes. In his absent-minded way, Leon loaded used paper in the photocopier and made another copy of his notes on clear plastic for the overhead projector. When he placed these two almost identical images in the folder he would use for his talk, all he saw was a single, smudgy-looking page. But when he laid the pages on his desk, one page happened to rotate a bit, and he noticed a pattern of circles emerging from the overlapping images.

Intrigued, Leon tried the process again. He took a blank sheet and copied it, getting black marks on the page. He set aside the original, copied the copy, and got a few more flecks on the resulting copy. After 10 cycles of copying, the paper was full of irregularly spaced black marks (Figure 4-1). Leon then placed the clear, plastic overhead on this paper, superimposing two copies of these thousands of black marks. Then he slowly rotated the overhead page until circles appeared. He took it further by enlarging the transparency. Superimposing the two, he now perceived radial lines. What was most odd is that there were no real lines on the page. Leon's brain abstracted these circles or radial lines from the pairs of images.[2]

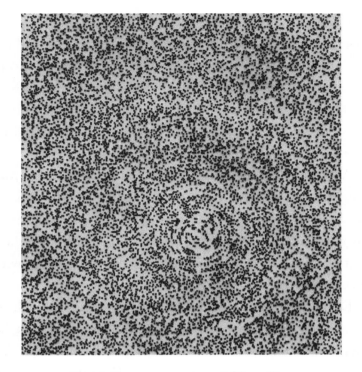

Fig. 4-I Glass pattern, courtesy of © Leon Glass.

Leon wondered whether color would alter these radial lines that he perceived. Not having color printers at his disposal in 1967, he learned silk screening, set up his dot patterns on a silk screen, and then printed them on paper. He printed one field of dots in yellow and one in blue. The circles vanished, making it clear that it was the "polarity" of the dots, not the color, that was important. White dots paired with black dots on a grey background did not work. The perceptual illusion fell apart.

In this same year, Hubel and Wiesel were just discovering orientation tuning and the functional architectures for which they would eventually win the Nobel Prize. The general understanding of the mechanics of vision was pretty thin. Leon knew that vision science should explain the radial lines, but when he got to McGill, no one was interested, and so these stimuli slept quietly unnoticed for almost ten years.

As an undergraduate at McGill, I heard about Glass's patterns firsthand when Leon told the copier story at a departmental seminar. I was fascinated both by Leon's simple way of telling the story and by the discovery itself. At around the time that Leon was telling us this story, his patterns were discovered by David Marr.

David Marr was one of the first modern neuroscience theorists. During his life, cut short at age thirty-five by leukemia, he laid out a program to understand the brain. His initial forays as a doctoral student at Cambridge in the late 1960s and early 1970s became a trio of singularly grand and complete theories of functions embodied in different parts of the brain. He explained how motor systems work,[3] how the cerebrum works, and how memory works. The titles of his papers were succinct: "A Theory of Cerebellar Cortex," "A Theory for Cerebral Neocortex," and "Simple Memory." Although these theoretical works have endured well over time, his last major work, a book called *Vision*, went well beyond them, setting the zeitgeist of brain science for the next twenty years.

In *Vision* Marr proposed that *definition* was the crucial neural problem to solve. Perhaps this simplification from complex mathematics to concepts it reflected was a realization that his previously published grand theories had been premature.[4] From the field of visual neuroscience, Marr selected a number of problems that could be defined well: Why did the world look three-dimensional from the images in our two eyes? How did we find the edges of objects? For each of these questions, he would lay out the computational problem, devise an algorithm to solve it (often culled from the scant biological experiments of the time), and provide a concrete expression of the steps needed to reach the solution.

Marr solved some of these more elementary problems. But the solutions to other problems were less clear. His book featured Leon Glass's random dot moiré patterns, presenting them as a perceptual illusion that required integrative features of the visual system as well as a challenge to be solved. So primed, visual psychophysicists began working in earnest with Glass patterns.

What fascinated me most about Leon's copier story was the idea of seeing something that was not actually there. The patterns could be very sparse (as they are in Figure 4-1), yet the circles were as clear as day. I knew of other optical illusions from grade school, such as the Müller-Lyer arrows that appeared to be different lengths but were not. Illusions of this sort were explained in terms of high-level cognitive function; for the

Müller-Lyer arrows, the explanation involved perspective and the corners of rooms. But Leon's patterns did not appear to have any high-level cognitive interpretation. You looked and out came circles or radial lines.

The patterns were also fascinating as a visual stimulus because they lacked all sorts of powerful standard visual cues; there were no lines, no colors. They spoke to me of the integrative power of the visual brain, a constructive ability to make order out of seeming chaos.

Simple ideas were proposed to explain the brain mechanisms that produce Glass patterns. A very quick-and-dirty approach to extract order from them was called "nearest neighbors." Take each point. When you find the point that is nearest to it, draw a line between the two points. Do this exhaustively for all the points. Then use some magic to connect all the pairs of line segments into shapes.

This approach is tedious—100 points produce about 10,000 pairs. What's worse is that the algorithm does not work at many levels. Depending on the number of points, the nearest-neighbor algorithm creates too many wrong matches. There is no obvious way to implement such an exhaustive search with neurons. And the joining of segments, even if they could be found, was a hack. One way around might be to call into play high-level cognitive processes. There also seem to be too many steps, with none of the fluidity of the real visual system. In fact, the game seems to fall into the trap that Edelman warns against—this problem is a world consisting of a tape of complex paired dots. However, our biological machine can solve the problem.

———

While most psychophysicists were ignoring Glass patterns, the biological machine was beginning to be understood. Hubel and Wiesel extracted many of the core principles of cortical organization. They understood that there was a map of the retina across the visual cortex, that each point in each eye had a portion of cortex dedicated to it. They found that the neurons in this portion of cortex were also tuned to specific characteristics of an image. The most salient, and so best described, image characteristic was orientation. Hubel and Wiesel examined the orientation selectivity of individual neurons by placing a small bar into a particular part of the visual world. If they hit the right part, the degree of the cell's excitation would be altered by the orientation of the bar.

It is an interesting coincidence that there was no room for any real "thinking" in these early measurements of the brain—indeed, the cats and monkeys used in these experiments were anesthetized. Visual stimuli came in through the eyes, and by the time they reached the cortex, the cortical machine had done its analysis, automatically measuring the orientation of each part of the image. The driving question of Hubel and Wiesel's time was how neurons became selective to orientation; their earliest models of orientation selectivity provided a hierarchical set of steps that built up more complex cells from simple components in a machine-like manner.

Through this research, Hubel and Wiesel found the hyper-column, a set of columns of neurons that systematically represents different orientations. These hypercolumns repeat, ultimately tiling the primary visual cortex with a cell for every location and every orientation.

This tiling of the cortex by orientation is the key to the biological interpretation of the Glass patterns. The visual cortex assesses the orientation at each location in the image. The beauty is that the neural circuitry that assesses these orientations does not need to make explicit judgments about the spacing between points. The result of this first stage of processing is a collection of neurons tiled across the cortical surface. Some are more acti-vated than others, depending on their selectivity to orientation and space and the registration between the pairs of dots.

As the Glass pattern has both local orientations that match the global percept and other orientations that do not, the result is an incomplete, ambiguous mapping that contains many of the elements of the global pattern, along with many spurious orien-tations. The final step here, similar to using the nearest-neighbor approach, is to match up the orientations that are close to each other and throw out the rest.

The neuroanatomists Kathleen S. Rockland and Jennifer S. Lund[5] laid out an ideal substrate to match up these nearby ori-entations. They injected small amounts of a tracer substance called horseradish peroxidase (HRP) into the visual cortex of the tree shrew, and found a beautiful latticework pattern run-ning across the cortical surface. Neurons were attached to neurons at long range—they could be separated by up to three millimeters, which is a huge distance in the cortex. (Rockland and Lund incorrectly hypothesized that these connections would be found in clumps, in which some portions of the cortex would have the long-range type and others would not.)

Rockland and Lund did correctly make a crucial inductive leap from their slides of fixed dead brain tissue. They suggested expanding Hubel and Wiesel's view of a visual cortex with repeated orientations to "the view of multiple repetitive structures intrinsic to the cortex, which may be adapted to fulfill a variety of functions." According to Lund's autobiographical notes,[6] for a short time, they thought they had found the holy grail of visual neuroscience: the structures that give rise to the orientation. But although they failed to find this grail, they had discovered something perhaps even more important.

Prior to publishing this work, Rockland and Lund shared their observations with Timothy Mitchison and Francis Crick, who suggested another function for the long-range connections: to connect similar orientations. If this were the case, it would mean that neurons with horizontal-orientation selectivity for one location in the visual world would communicate with neurons that selected this same orientation but for a different location. This ingenious circuit could then be used to form complex properties of neuronal receptive fields. Like Rockland and Lund, Mitchison and Crick were partly wrong in that they predicted additional properties of the long-range connections that subsequent anatomical study did not confirm. Yet as a small explosion of work on these horizontal connections established, Mitchison and Crick's purely theoretical analysis was absolutely correct in one essential aspect: like did talk to like. Although Rockland and Lund missed the "like-to-like" possibility, they were right that these connections could be adapted to fulfill "a variety of functions."

One of these functions is the perceiving of Glass patterns. In those patterns, a local orientation measurement has a certain possibility of fitting into the global percept, the image being observed, and a certain possibility of not fitting. The long-range connections provide a substrate for nearby orientation measurements to influence each other. As a result, if the orientations at two nearby locations are similar, the long-range connections permit them to connect with each other and be mutually supportive, but if the two orientations are very different, the cells will not connect with and support each other. Thus, rough colinearity of orientation across the image can be established.

This computational approach to the perceiving of Glass patterns came from an unlikely corner of computer vision: Steven Zucker, then at McGill University. Zucker was one of the earliest researchers outside of David Marr's MIT Vision Group to pay close attention to the biological substrates that could solve really hard perceptual problems. He designed a computer algorithm that propagated local orientation information across the image. For reasons that remain obscure, it was called relaxation labeling.[7] Zucker tested his algorithm with Glass patterns. Working with constraints on the number of points and the spacing between points,[8] he was able to demonstrate that such a biologically inspired algorithm could *perceive* these patterns.

Glass patterns are an abstraction of natural textures that are amenable to scientific examination. David Marr held them up as a looking glass from the real world that would help vision scientists carefully consider what it means to perceive. The world is full of all sorts of textures at so many different scales—trees covering a hillside, the grain of wood, the warp and weft of cloth, sheaves of wheat in a field, fine eyelashes on a model. Marr knew it would be very hard in 1982 to biologically test and to come up with computational algorithms to perceive all of these things. And indeed, there has been a broadening of perceptual science as we pass into the looking glass of the abstracted world, with increased biologically inspired implementations.[9] The Glass patterns are now a hard mark in the vision field.

FIVE

BRIGHT MOMENTS

I n the mid-1980s, William Newsome, Anthony Movshon, and Kenneth Britten (Newsome's postdoctoral fellow) published a series of papers that I consider to be seminal. They asked how many neurons were needed to encode a particular perceptual decision. Is one neuron enough, or do you need a group of neurons in order to tell yourself what you see?

This study was the culmination of an effort to relate a neuron's activity directly to an internal percept. In 1972, the psychologist Horace Barlow wrote a paper that was way ahead of its time in many ways, titled "Single units and sensation: A neuron doctrine for perceptual psychology?" Note the question mark at the end of the title. The very first sentence clearly and painfully lays out the problem: "In this article I shall discuss the difficult but challenging problem of the relation between our subjective perceptions and the activity of the nerve cells in our brains."

This is all there is to it. All cortical neuroscientists need to do is answer this simple question of how neurons relate to what we see.

Barlow distilled his argument to five dogmas, five imperious dogmas:[1]

1. To understand nervous function one needs to look at interactions at a cellular level, rather than either a more macroscopic or microscopic level, because behaviour depends upon the organized pattern of these intercellular interactions.

2. The sensory system is organized to achieve as complete a representation of the sensory stimulus as possible with the minimum number of active neurons.

3. Trigger features of sensory neurons are matched to redundant patterns of stimulation by experience, as well as by developmental processes.

4. Perception corresponds to the activity of a small selection from the very numerous high-level neurons, each of which corresponds to a pattern of external events of the order of complexity of the events symbolized by a word.

5. High impulse frequency in such neurons corresponds to high certainty that the trigger feature is present.

The plan was clear. Psychologists needed to stop looking at phenomena and start looking at neurons. Barlow saw the brain as a group of mostly silent-yet-smart neurons; when a neuron had something important to say, it would shout it out with lots of activity, with "high-impulse frequency." When the specialized "high-level" neurons were active, we perceived.

Barlow got some of the details wrong: many neurons are active at once, and specialized high-level neurons that match up to our percept do not exist. But his work called upon psychologists to look directly at both what physiologists were doing and the details of the circuits.

How was one to make these direct brain/behavior comparisons in a human or nonhuman primate? The neurophysiologists knew what to do and were already hard at work. Vernon Mountcastle realized early on that it was crucial to directly compare the neurons' tuning properties to what the animal reported seeing. But in 1968,[2] it was technically beyond Mountcastle's capability to ask a monkey what it perceived while recording what its neurons were doing. So he and his group assumed that monkeys and humans had the same perceptions and split the experiment between the two.

In their experiments, the human participants reported by pushing a button when they felt a vibratory flutter stimulus on the palms of their hands. The strength of the flutter would vary. For flutters too weak to feel, the participant would feel nothing and not push the button; for strong flutters, the participant would always push the button; for intermediate flutters, the participant might push the button. A psychometric function, which is a graph of the amplitude of the vibration versus the button pushes, shows quantitatively how much vibration is needed for the human subject to perceive it.

Mountcastle took these techniques, which were well understood, commonly used, and noncontroversial in the study of humans, and used the same equipment and protocols to study monkeys. He took recordings from single nerve fibers in the hand of the anesthetized monkey, and then in the primary somatosensory cortex of the post-central gyrus of unanesthetized awake monkeys.

Since Mountcastle assumed that the human participants' psychometric function was identical to metrics derived from the monkey, if he could assess the neural events in the monkey, it would be as if he knew the neural events in the human, and so could find out whether the mental event, the perception, was identical with the firing of the neuron.

To explore this identity question, the humans' behavior and the neurons' activity needed to be compared on the same playing field. Using ideal observer theory, Mountcastle's group constructed a quantitative encoding of the human behavioral data called the receiver-operator characteristic (ROC). They defined a neural code. The number crunching indeed revealed a degree of match between the dependence of the brain's code and the human discrimination.[3]

These studies had two key flaws. First, human data were compared with monkey data. Second, the monkey was not performing any task during the neural assessment. Despite the elegance of these studies, they had failed to record cells during the monkeys' perceptions.

But by the mid-1980s, Mountcastle's pioneering studies with Edward Evarts had turned from the early somatosensory cortex to the inferior parietal lobule, in which so many secrets of higher perception appeared to hide.

Laboratories grew from these two main branches of Evarts and Mountcastle. People such as Charles Gross brought on younger scientists to start on the somewhat simpler problem of motion perception: Which neurons in our brains are responsible for conveying that something moved? Along with Tom Albright, Gross found that an area called MT (named for the middle temporal region in a New World monkey) has a map, a representation of motion, that is architecturally similar to the representations of orientation and eye dominance in nearby V I. Pieces of cortex represent pieces of the world, and even more important, there are isolated segments of the cortex for every movement direction. Through the work of Albright, Gross, and many others, MT became the next big thing, the place to go to find out whether the neuron carried the percept.

William Newsome was another who found a path to follow from the Barlow and Mountcastle studies. He and Robert Wurtz wanted to find out whether highly focused lesions in the Old World monkey's MT could remove a tiny portion of visual experience. Enough was known about the cortex's organization, connections, and role in perception for them to point directly at MT, manipulate it, and presume what would happen. They trained monkeys to perform psychophysical visual-motion experiments, and created small chemical lesions in the motion area MT that made the monkeys motion-blind.

Newsome began to work on the big problem—both experimentally and conceptually—of matching perception and neuronal activity. The initial experimental steps were straightforward enough. He would do both parts of Mountcastle's study in the same animal. He trained monkeys to use eye movements to indicate the direction of dots' motion on a screen. He altered the amount of motion so that gauging the motion's direction was impossible under some conditions and easy under others. From these data, he could compute psychometric functions. While the monkey was doing this, neurons were recorded from the motion area MT. The hard part, as it had been for Mountcastle, was finding a level playing field for comparing the monkey's percept and the signaling of the neurons.

Mountcastle had brought forward an idea. Tony Movshon provided the means to make the dream into reality by applying a precise recipe from signal-detection theory to neural activity and deriving a "neurometric" function to match up with the behaviorally based psychometric function.

In 1986, at the annual Society for Neuroscience meeting, Newsome presented the physiological and behavioral data in the first of two radical platform talks. In the second, Ken Britten presented the neurometric results.

I remember few—if any—questions after the second talk. It was too new and different. I, at least, was dumbfounded. I went up to Newsome in the hallway later, and before I could say anything, he asked me, "Did anyone understand what we said?"

In time we understood. The Newsome, Britten, and Movshon study[4] presented a monkey with a simple perceptual task and recorded from single neurons in the motion area MT. Common sense would say that one neuron is not equal to your perception: blow out one neuron and you still see. Instead they found that a single cell behaved as well as the entire animal. This joint neurometric and psychometric analysis says that, given a particular choice, the single neuron and the monkey are equally smart. The single-neuron-equals-a-percept idea became part of the canon. The years pass, and an idea, once new, if good, remains.

In the mid-1990s, Tom Albright and I were discussing this result. Tom noted that Simona Celebrini and Newsome had observed that the match of psychophysical and neuronal thresholds is also similar for the medial superior temporal area (MST), an area that receives the output of the early motion area MT. MST also processes motion, but it has neurons that report more complex motions, such as those occurring as we navigate the world.

Tom pointed out that although the single-neuron-equals-a-percept idea was true for MT, it was not clear whether it was true for MST. What was wrong? He also wondered whether the difficulty of the task mattered. Perhaps one neuron could easily represent a binary choice—is the motion going left or right?—but it might falter when more complexity and subtlety were needed. What do more complexity and subtlety mean for a monkey? Perhaps choosing one of five directions was a sufficiently more complex test. Might a complex task require more neurons?

And suddenly the entire conversation, the entire moment becomes clear in my memory. I was visiting Tom and his wife Lisa back in 1994 in their house in Leucadia, not far from the San Diego Botanic Garden, surrounded by dozens of cycads. We were sitting, all three of us, on a couch in the darkly wooded den. Lisa had fallen asleep. In the drowsy world of late night talks, we discussed these new results—neurons, ROC curves, monkey psychophysics, choice probabilities. The evening darkened about us. Lisa remained silently asleep—presumably Tom's and my conversation was not the most scintillating. A so-strong remembrance fills me. Tom is picking Lisa up in his arms, a tiny bundle, and carrying her gently off to bed. The palpable love of that moment, the utter trust urgently resounding in the quiet of the moment, etched itself onto my neurons for remembrance now. How many neurons—what choice probabilities—of that encoding led back to this moment? It took only a single neuron loaded with synaptic strengths in its dendrites, pregnant with potentiality and actualized ideas, to recall the perfect moment of Tom and Lisa.

SIX

EIGHTH AVENUE LINE AT FOURTEENTH STREET

Oliver Sacks is working on an essay about time.[1] Toward the end of the draft, he started talking about foamy time, a concept in quantum mechanics. I suggested that he would be better off talking about neurological time. We stopped at the Fourteenth Street entrance to the Eighth Avenue subway line. It had been an exhilarating day; we had been talking non-stop about almost everything. I wanted to stay and clarify time; I had to go; I was caught in a singularity of time.

How is time encoded? What is the meaning of "now"? These have been questions that I have heard of, thought of, and sometimes even worked on. I had always enjoyed space-time representations in special relativity classes. Space and time, Einstein showed, were equivalent dimensions $[x, y, z, ct]$.

Four-dimensional space. It was easily perceivable, tangible, and graphable. It was straightforward physics.

Physiological time was another matter. I had never thought of the "now" in biological terms until I heard Francis Crick musing about it back in 1984 at David Rumelhart's weekly PDP (Parallel Distributed Processing) Research Group. Dick Birks, whose McGill laboratory I had worked in, specialized in mechanisms of short-term retention of memory. He favored posttetanic potentiation (PTP). That is, if you electrically blast (tetanize) a synapse for five seconds with thirty stimuli per second, the synapse will become augmented at two time scales. The intense augmentation lasts less than half a second; a weaker form persists for half a minute.

At Rumelhart's weekly meeting, Francis Crick wondered what biological mechanism corresponded to the "now." We all knew, he said, that the "now" was less than one second. Did he ask, did he say, did I answer "PTP"? He asked whether anyone had studied PTP or long-term potentiation (LTP) in the cortex. Could the timing of PTP parallel the timing of, and also be the source of, the "now"?

I took it upon myself to call Tim Bliss—who had first reported the longer memory mechanism LTP in the hippocampus. (I had a tenuous connection; Bliss was once Dick Birks' graduate student.) He did not know of anyone doing these measurements in cortex. I looked online.[2] The NIH database, Medline, revealed only two papers on LTP in cortex: one in dentate cortex, and one from a Russian group, unread

I was sure.[3] I passed these on to Francis, and both of us went on to other things. Over the years, I continued to pursue time with my chaos theory of brain, and Francis continued to chase the "now" through his exploration of consciousness with Christof Koch and others.

Fast-forward seventeen years to my sabbatical at the Salk. Francis has reasserted himself on the question of physiological time. I am staring at the ocean from my aerie. Oliver Sacks is finishing another book, *Uncle Tungsten*. I go to the Helmholtz Club, for the first time since my postdoctoral studies.

The Helmholtz Club had been initiated by Francis Crick to bring together the best vision scientists in Southern California. Each month, the club met at UC Irvine. The members were all at the top of their field—John Allman, David Van Essen, Joseph Bogen, V. S. Ramachandran, Richard Andersen, David Rumelhart. Francis would select two speakers and the group would pore over a vision problem. It was considered an honor to attend as a postdoctoral trainee; you only got to go if the material was your specialty. I had been lucky enough to be invited twice. We drove up to Irvine. Lunch first; I sat across from David Van Essen for the first time, staring at him in awe. He had laid out the circuitry of MT, and the inputs gave him the clues he needed to form the circuits. Each lecture was allotted two hours; each slide, each detail was pulled apart, dissected, and critiqued. Afterwards, the group of twenty went out for dinner, discussion continuing well into the evening. I went home exhausted and happy.

At lunch with David Eagleman and me, Francis is thinking aloud about wagon-wheel illusions and stable configurations of neurons. The "wagon-wheel illusion" is named after the odd ways that the wheels of a Conestoga wagon appear in Western movies. Although the wagon is moving forward, the wheels appear to stop or rotate backward. This is because its spokes are caught in only brief periods of time by the twenty-four-frames-per-second movie film. If the wheel is moving at just the right speed, the visual pictures on the film actually represent a wheel running backward. Leon Glass, a Mathematical Master of Chaos, had pursued this illusion.

But the wagon-wheel illusion that Francis and David are going on about is a bit different. Apparently it can be observed in daylight. Lying on your back, staring at a rapidly spinning fan over your bed, you may perceive that the fan blades spontaneously change direction.

As there is no external strobe, Francis and David reasoned, the strobe must be in your mind. Something is clocking the neurons in and out of sync. I have an almost visible picture of neurons flickering in and out of coherent groups. Perhaps some cell is leading them—"one cell to rule them all and in the darkness bind them." Or perhaps there is a more cooperative phenomenon.

As I listen at lunch my mind rushes through the dynamics of cortex I have been thinking about. So many parts are coming together: chaos, my graduate work on synaptic plasticity, the "now," perceptual illusions, and self-organizing visual cortex.

Indeed years earlier, I had proposed this study to NIH. Part of the project was to examine how neuronal populations entrain to temporally bistable illusions of rotating plates,[4] and part was to model populations of neurons. Would the actual neurons lock into bistable patterns? My proposal remained unfunded, so I never found out.

And now it is back to the Eighth Avenue station with Oliver. There are just a few moments to deliver this "package of time." I must have been clear enough, because the next time we speak, his essay is now pondering all the parts of biological and neurological time.

Oliver describes Necker cubes reversing and demands to know more about my bald assertion that the "now" is 350 milliseconds long. Can the shortness of the "now" explain the Necker cubes? At the moment, I have no answer. But his time scales are too long: Necker cube reversals take seconds, and the "now" lasts 350 milliseconds and changes at 3 hertz.

I do have an entire set of illusions that have a strong 3 Hz component. They include *The Enigma* by Isia Leviant, which Torsten Wiesel placed by the elevator at his laboratory at Rockefeller, so his scientists would contemplate it and marvel at how little we could explain (Figure 6-1). David Marr's examples of flickering grouping dots and the famous scintillating grid illusion also have this persistent beat (Figure 6-2),[5] as do migraine auras.[6] Could the source be PTP? Bringing neurons together and apart at 3 Hz would be the role of this biological short-term-memory phenomenon. Indeed, PTP might not even

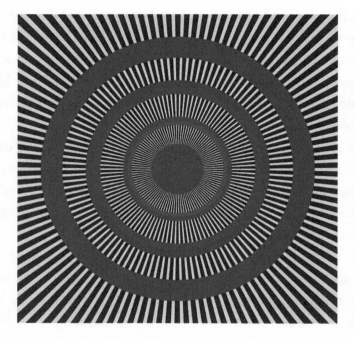

Fig. 6-1 Scientists at Torsten Wiesel's neurobiology laboratory stared at
this three-foot-wide image for a few minutes each day, while waiting
for the elevator. How did it spin, and what was Torsten's point
in placing it there?

have a critical role in memory, but might instead be the basis of
the biological "now."

I must lay out this simplistic hypothesis, knowing full well
that the mathematics inherent in such a complex neural system
might prove me wrong.

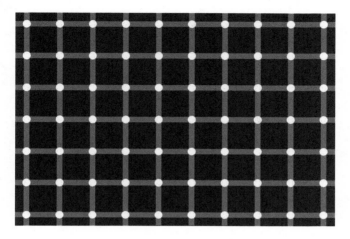

Fig. 6-2 Scintillating grid illusion. Courtesy of Bernd Lingelbach.

SEVEN

MODERN TIMES

A Computational Neurobiology Laboratory journal club meeting was being held at ten o'clock, smack dab in the middle of my sabbatical writing time. I dawdled, but eventually got myself there. As I go into the room, I see an overhead transparency projected on the wall—very few people are using overheads any more. And then I see Terry Sejnowski presenting the paper.

Now, Terry has been in neuroscience since I was in high school, yet still maintains a youthful enthusiasm. He is part and parcel of the neuroscience community here.

I first heard of him when he invented Net-Talk. I was a fresh young postdoctoral fellow excited to be invited for Sunday dinner at Odile and Francis Crick's house. I heard the edge of a conversation. On the *Good Morning America* television show in 1985, someone played a tape of a computer learning to talk. First the computer babbled; then it started to speak more realistically.

A short while later, Terry came to talk at the Parallel Computing Group meeting across the street from the Salk at UCSD. All the greats-to-be were there: Rumelhart, Zipser, McClelland, Crick, Andersen, Asanuma, and a host of others whose names I did not know or have forgotten. Terry presented his Net-Talk. The idea was simple—to get a machine to translate written text to phonemes.

A model was constructed with three layers. The input was the text; the output, the phonemes. The network was trained to find relationships between the two, using a numerical technique called "backprop."[1] The three-layer network architecture in itself was not amazing. The power of the model was in the non-linearities of the connections between the layers. Repeated presentations of training material taught the network to find better and better relationships between the written text and the phonemes—just like a child learning to read out loud. All this was done on a computer, with the text and phonemes encoded as binary strings of ones and zeros.

Terry did something special. Instead of just looking at the numbers, he attached the model's digital output to a Digital Equipment Company phoneme-to-sound decoder and recorded the result on a cassette tape. When Net-Talk was stupid and taught nothing, the train of phonemes were not matched correctly to the input words and it sounded like babble. But after Net-Talk was trained, any talk show host could hear the changes wrought in the model. It became intelligible.

And beyond the Net-Talk idea itself, and the making of a cassette tape that could be played on *Good Morning America*, Terry had a third stroke of genius made transparently obvious by a simple question.

A longhaired faculty member, who seemed a bit put out by the whole hurrah, asked, "Did you choose the childlike voice for the phoneme translator?"

Terry packaged the entire product in a way to appeal to all of us. He could have chosen a gruff basso voice, but the innocence of the child lured and seduced us. Like Humbert Humbert we were taken to our desires. A waif backed by a most powerful computer.

So in I walk—twenty minutes late. It is traditional for graduate students and postdoctoral trainees to speak at these meetings, and so I am surprised that Terry is speaking. The only seat is right in front of him, so off I go. It is a very technical background paper that is presented journal-club style. It was obvious that he knew the gist of the paper, but he was also thinking on his feet. (I, too, like to give informal talks not fully ready. It adds an edge and adrenaline to the situation.)

His second figure had six panels; it was complicated. The paper was a fourth-order story about long-term potentiation (LTP). Most often studied in the hippocampus, LTP is a process that electrically assesses the activity across a synapse.

One stimulates the input to a cell and watches the postsynaptic potential (PSP). A burst of input or some other manipulation occurs, and the PSP will increase or decrease for hours. It is the most cellular substantiation of what we all think of as memory and learning.

But the odd thing, known from the first extracellular recordings of Bliss and Lomo in 1973, is that the signal contains an incredible amount of noise. Many researchers have spent years—even entire careers—trying to understand LTP or LTD (long-term depression).[2] Most of them simply average out the noise—ignoring variability—the most conspicuous message.

The actual meat of the paper was quite esoteric, but Terry presented it to challenge each of us there to question. He is very good at tying the issues back to ongoing work in his group.

Toward the end of the journal club, the question of noise in the postsynaptic potential came up—what was its purpose? Ideas were floated about noise's role in synaptic communication, following the argument of Terry's study.

I had a question outside the paper's intent and unrelated to most of what had come before. I expected to hear either a "No" or more vague speculation. But I pushed ahead anyway. For after all, isn't that what a sabbatical is all about? Pushing oneself and others to go a bit beyond the beaten path.

"Are there any computational models that *exploit* the noise?"

Terry Sejnowski reaches deep into his intellectual back pocket and says, "There was a paper—rarely cited—that was written a while ago, 1995, in *Network*.[3] It was one of the very best on the subject." Smiling mischievously, he continued, "It had been written by me." That paper was a model of integrate-and-fire neurons, which thrive on noise. He had interconnected them in a model of brain tissue to see what happened at the "thermodynamic limit."

As you approach the thermodynamic limit in modeling, you typically increase the number of particles in a simulation and watch the behavior smooth out from random to predictable. Individual gas molecules are noisy, unpredictable little brats, but put together you have a well-behaved crowd. For example, if you could watch the individual particles of diatomic oxygen, carbon dioxide, and nitrogen in air through a super-microscope, you could never guess which way each particle would go next. But these gas molecules behave well in large numbers. If you consider air in a child's balloon, you know that when you open the nozzle, air will rush out in a wholly predictable way. Mathematically this is done by increasing the number of particles in a simulation and watching the behavior smooth out from random to predictable—the thermodynamic limit.

Terry put together large numbers of these noisy integrate-and-fire neurons, but he didn't take the typical approach of smoothing out the behavior. Instead he forced the system of neurons to increase the noise as he increased the number of synapses. In doing so, he created a system that was stable but could easily move from one behavior to another. It was as if the well-behaved crowd of thousands could start singing the "Star Spangled Banner," then instantly and effortlessly switch to "I've

Got a Lovely Bunch of Coconuts," then to "God Save the Queen." The system of neurons had become supple.

"Perhaps that is what creativity is," Terry said. "There are two competing noisy inputs to a noisy-but-well-behaved crowd of cells. And the crowd jumps to a new state. Aha! A new idea!"

Terry's idea of noisy synapses permitting such switching was indeed novel and certainly resonated with everyone. Terry then mentioned a meeting in which he and an experimentalist, Haim Sompolinsky, first discussed this idea. Sompolinsky argued against it, asserting that noisy neurons could not switch quickly. Terry thought that was the end of the conversation until six months later, when Sompolinsky published a modeling study showing rapid switching in noisy chaotic networks.[4]

One of the scientists around the table asked what Terry thought of this turn of events.

"We learn from our mistakes," he said.

Wanting to get a last word in, I said, "Perhaps it was a success," which earned me a wry smile.

On the drive to work this morning along the Del Mar coast, I told Jasmine, my wife, about this. She said noise had altered her creativity yesterday on the beach. The sounds of the ocean on the rocks at Torrey Pines Beach, the different colors, the lighting, the ocean had given her raw materials to rapidly combine to new creative thoughts. She was doing this at the same moment I was with Terry. She remarked, "Maybe it is something in the air here." And indeed it is.

EIGHT

VISUAL IRREDENTISM

Irredentism: The policy or programme of the Irredentists. Also in extended use: any policy of seeking the recovery and reunion to one country of a region or regions for the time being subject to another country. (*Oxford English Dictionary*)

In the mid-twelfth century a small but powerful group headed north to claim the Austrian Alps for Italy. They settled in, and seven centuries later, irredentism was born as a movement to claim for Italy the Tyrolean Alps, to join the brothers, sisters, cousins, aunts, and uncles who shared their common cultural and historical bonds, ultimately forming a Grande Italia. *Italia irredenta* failed, however, because living in the Alps free of Papal rule was simply too appealing to the Tyroleans. Yet the urge to join up with people estranged by the vagaries of political, historical, or geographical boundaries remains strong, and so the world continues to be wracked by conflicts of modern day irredentists. Such tensions resolve when the boundaries are dissolved by communication, as happened in 1989 when the Berlin Wall fell. Our brain's cortices, thalamic nuclei, and brainstem structures seem destined to share this fate.

For many reasons, we brain scientists believe that the subdivisions into which we have divided the brain should functionally join into a cooperative, holistic worldview. We know that we form our conscious perception of the world by fusing disparate parts of our representations of it into a coherent whole—this is referred to as the binding problem. During the past decade or two, a major goal of cortical neuroscience has been to find a neural substrate to support this fusing of disparate representations.

When I began my postdoctoral training at the Salk Institute, I joined a weekly journal club, a small, intimate group in which we would present current papers or hear guest speakers. Francis Crick would attend, which thrilled my young postdoctoral self.

One guest speaker was Christoph von der Malsburg. I knew nothing of him, his work, or the problems he was scrutinizing. There were eight of us and a blackboard. He spoke about the oddest topic: cocktail parties. His story went roughly that when you are at cocktail party, you hear a constant stream of multiple conversations. You can effortlessly listen to one voice among the many. How? He then spoke of modeling collections of neurons that were bound together through an oscillation. The "knowledge" that would be encoded by the system would be in the strengths of its connections.

His idea sounded really strange to me because, at first, it seemed to have absolutely nothing to do with the visual system I was studying. We were working with what Malsburg called a "conventional brain theory." According to this theory, neurons could encode certain things, such as a color. These neurons were organized across the cortex in a way that their physical location matched up with the thing being encoded. To perceive was to have the correct set of neurons activated. Malsburg described how this theory saw the brain as a projection screen.

Indeed, that was my research project at the time. I wanted to know how neurons in the parietal cortex flashed on and off as a monkey looked around. How was the location of objects in the world linked to the flashing of neurons on the "projection screen" of the cortex?

Malsburg went on and on, using words such as oscillations, synchrony, correlation, and binding, and writing equations with a term "w_{ij}," that stood for synaptic strength (weight). He thought it was essential that the connection between neurons could change rapidly.

The "projection-screen view" had unchanging synaptic strengths. I knew that changing synaptic strength changed the input to a neuron. How could my parietal neurons have different synaptic strengths, different inputs each day, and still indicate the same thing? Malsburg's view was of neurons that oscillated in synchrony, forming vast spatial and temporal structures at multiple scales in the cortex.

Although I understood oscillators and attractor theory, the biology that Malsburg spoke of was like a foreign language. He said he was talking about the cortex and pulling disparate threads of processing together. He had laid out many of the principles, starting almost from the first ones, those that have occupied neuroscience for twenty years. He presented this work in what Francis Crick called "the most obscure paper in science"—its prescience was remarkable.[1]

At the time, I had no idea what I was hearing, no idea that a shift was occurring from looking at the brain as a screen to looking at it as an active and flexible participant in generating our internal state. I had no idea of the ferment around me. I simply thought these ideas made sense and were the natural progression. I was surrounded by exceedingly bright scientists and their ideas washed over me, permeated me. I had no concept that I was living in a particularly exciting time.

Over the next few years, experimental studies confirmed and explored Malsburg's ideas. Perhaps the most important of these was a study done in 1989 by Charles Gray and Wolf Singer, which I first saw as a preprint forwarded by Crick.[2] Their studies in cats found electrical fields in the cortex oscillating at forty times per second. Gray and Singer claimed that these oscillations arose from masses of neurons firing in synchrony—exactly one of the predictions of Malsburg's theoretical effort.

Gray and Singer expanded on this idea by asserting that these oscillations were found whenever two elements needed to be bound together, challenging the primary visual cortex with stimuli that needed to be integrated—*bound together*—to be perceived. At an annual meeting of the Society for Neuroscience in 1990, it was standing room only as Singer presented his latest results.

Singer reasoned that when you saw a red ball rolling across the green grass, parts of your brain were activated by the red, parts by the ball, parts by the grass, and parts by the motion. However, you don't see the world in these individual parts but as a single, coherent whole. And of course, as noted earlier in this chapter, how it is all brought together—*bound together*—is the binding problem.

I had always thought that Malsburg had originated the phrase, "binding problem," but he does not even mention the word "binding" until a 1985 paper.[3] Gray and Singer do not mention the phrase in their early work. Although Anne Treisman started using the term in her publications during the 1990s, she has told me she is not its originator. It seems that the term and the role of oscillations emerged spontaneously from Malsburg's foundational concepts. A major change had occurred in how we thought about a core problem.

What made the role of oscillations and binding so relevant was that it was the beginning of a physiology that moved beyond descriptions of filtered neurons. These were active elements that interacted with each other to cause oscillations. Areas were bringing each other into the fold of the coherent unitary percept. Neurons had become irredentists.

The neuroscience of vision has been extremely successful—the visual system is certainly the best understood of the senses. And in our glory, we reach out to enjoin other cortices, other thalamic nuclei, and other brainstem structures to be part of our grand catholic vision. Those confused neurons in the valleys of orbital cortex and the highlands of premotor must be brought home.

It is not clear who our pope is, but we certainly have more than our share of cardinals. Cardinals David Van Essen and Daniel Felleman have been our cartographers, neatly drawing a nexus of crossing lines, right angles, binding together dozens of cortical areas. Cardinal Charlie Gross has forced us out into new lands, using the sharp end of a stick, the microelectrode, to place flags further and further away from the homeland of the eye.

Still for all of our land grabs—these are indeed conquests—we find the whole is still made up of many parts. Are we visual imperialists, who impose our will onto new parts of the brain? Or are we visual irredentists, who see the patch of premotor cortex not as a foreign territory but as a place closely linked to the visual system?

Under a microscope, the local circuits and cell types of the classically studied visual area in the superior temporal cortical area do not look all that different from those of the premotor cortex. Neurons in both cortices happily respond to visual stimuli—in the premotor cortex, you simply have to embed the stimuli into the right behavioral sequence. The two cortices even speak the same language; the same neural code is embedded in the action potentials. Listening in on neurons with a sharp electrode, the sound is the same regardless of the area being pierced. These areas are simply segregated by the politics of the early historical successes of one of the sensory sciences, by the politics of funding, and by the geography of the sulci and gyri.

Today, there are two levels to our vision science. The first level is the analysis of neurons and areas, dealing with the properties of each area as a separate entity, as an independent scientific problem. Even though we know neurons and areas are not independent, we plan our experiments as if they were. We may combine a motor property or one or more visual properties into the task performed by the animal, but ultimately we ask how that one area can provide a combinatorial representation. Sometimes we try to find out how they interact, perhaps assuming they must interact, but no great successes have revolutionized our study of the brain. Sorting out these properties is an enormous creative effort, with the visual imperialists finding the most esoteric properties combined with vision.

The second level of analysis is a stratification of the responses of these areas into a visual hierarchy, into one culture of a visually inspired brain. Anatomical projections are used as guide and constraint. Highly satisfying maps and theories have emerged to explain the first steps of the visual processing of color and motion.

Still, progress has been slow, and it remains hard to see how all of these disparate lands can be bound together. The cocktail party problem and oscillations did not provide the solution, although they have sent visual neuroscience in diverse directions. Perhaps the culture that served us so admirably during the first steps of visual neuroscience may fail to bring together the remote cortices. Perhaps it needs to be discarded.

Does the replacement theory lie ahead of us, or does it lie already discovered and ignored in the Alpine crevasses? In 1978, Vernon Mountcastle and Gerald Edelman coauthored a perfect little book called *The Mindful Brain*.[4] Each wrote succinctly on his passion for cortical organization.

Mountcastle, in the midst of his furthest expeditions into cognition and associational cortices, described the anatomical basis of the cortical columns—the representational elements that we know, years later, still need to be bound together. Edelman marched forth with his new selectionist theory of cortical function, derived in part from his immunological canon and Darwin's theory of natural selection. Both provide missing elements for the solution of the binding problem, but if they were not ignored, they certainly had not reached the collective unconscious of visual neuroscience by the mid-1980s.

Edelman's passion centers on a competition. Neurons discover their meanings through constant interaction and rediscovery of relationships. Could this be the mechanism that our visual system uses to dynamically bind similar stuff in the incoming sensorium into a coherent singular percept?[5] Neurons and groups of neurons compete with each other for synaptic resources, much as the Tyroleans and the Papists fought over acreage. For the irredentists, the answer was the final status of their states, not as decided by a pope, but by a war. For neurons too, there is no "decider," no pope instructing his vassals how to distribute territory. Edelman[6] lets the brain sort out its own territory, using "reentry," a conversation between neurons and assemblies, to select and bind the correct surviving groups, the new political topography—the new political order.

The irredentists are all but forgotten. Tyrol is still in the Alps and the Tyroleans share some common ancestry and some recognizable traits with Italians; yet they have remained distinct and independent from Italy. Can one posit—and then confirm—a theory of brain function that allows such weak links to remain, providing for commerce over borders and peaceful coexistence, yet where the tensions between the separated regions are a source of powerful neural computation, and so a mature science of the mind?

NINE

CRITIQUE OF PURE CORTICAL TOPOGRAPHY

One key principle used to unlock the function of cerebral cortex is that of the map. A map refers to the orderly progression of some feature across the cortical surface. This principle arises from the orderly input of the external world upon our sensorium. For example, the image on the retina has a natural mapping onto the cortical sheet of early visual cortex. In his 1944 Ferrier Lecture to the Royal Society, Gordon Holmes reported that by analyzing shrapnel punctures in a soldier's cortex, he was able to map locations in the visual field to particular physical spots in the visual cortex (Figure 9-I).[1] He concluded, "It has been possible to construct a map of the visual cortex on which the cortical area related to each segment of the retina can be shown."

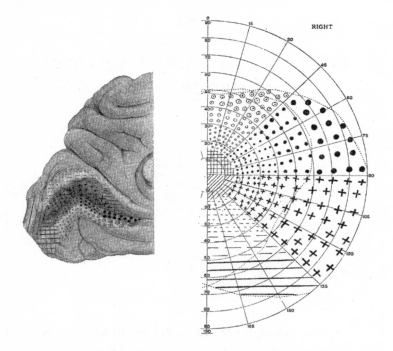

Fig. 9-1 The representation of the primary visual cortex. The diagram
to the left shows the middle of the rear cortex. To its right is a map of
the retinotopy found from bullets and shrapnel that had penetrated
the cortex. Reprinted from Gordon Holmes, "Ferrier Lecture:
The Organization of the Visual Cortex in Man," Figure 5/ page 352,
1945, *The Royal Society*. Used with kind permission of The Royal Society.

This is also true for our skin. Different neurons fire
when each finger is touched; the finger "touch" neurons are
organized across the somatosensory cortex in a hand-like pattern (Figure 9-2). Cortex mathematically almost matches the
inputs from our senses.

Sensory   Motor

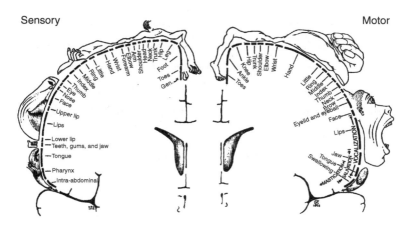

Fig. 9-2 Two regions of cortex that contain sensory and motor representations. Reprinted from W. Penfield and T. Rasmussen, *The Cerebral Cortex of
Man.* © 1950 Gale, a part of Cengage Learning, Inc. Reproduced by
permission. www.cengage.com/permissions.

For example, within a very good approximation, a blue light
of a certain brightness leads to the same response in the retinal
ganglion cells that transmit the signal to the relay stations of the
thalamus and then onto the visual cortex. Each of them has a
place mapping, which means that cells near each other in the
thalamus or the cortex reflect proximity in real places in the
world. Other properties are also embedded within these retinotopic maps. This is what led Hubel and Wiesel to propose the
idea of the functional architecture. In their 1971 Ferrier Lecture,
they demarcated a whole series of mappings in the visual primary
cortex, yet it is striking that a careful reading of the lecture fails
to reveal a strict definition of the term "functional architecture."[2]
Each reader, nonetheless, understands exactly what it is.

The way that touch, light, and sound sensors strike our sensorium is certainly constant; the physical properties of light do not change. And in the absence of severe perturbations,[3] it follows that the primary representations of the external world also remain constant across time, through the processing of the cortex.

These ideas of constant sensory representations give rise to the idea that the internal cortical representations are fixed and hard wired. When we think of some abstract idea such as a mathematical formulation of the origins of the universe, a Chopin mazurka, or love, the extension of the idea of consistent sensory representation leads us to believe that a particular area of the brain lights up, is activated. That concept is deeply embedded in our science. These ideas of fixity of brain mappings have become an archetype for the public's view of the brain. Beautiful functional brain images published in the *New York Times* and *Scientific American* show hot orange patches that are our minds.

According to this way of thinking, not only is the entire area switching on when you think of a walk taken in the woods last year, but particular groups of neurons also consistently represent that walk. A map somewhere in your brain collects neurons for each event, each idea, each concept. This makes the idea of programming the brain simple. Each area takes the signals from a map or collection of maps and synthesizes a new map.

We neuroscientists have been terribly wrong. We relied a bit too much on what we thought we knew. What really matters is not what is outside, but what is inside. And what is inside is constantly changing. My own work forced me to this conclusion. Experiments that examined the representations of motion and objects' location in the world drove us crazy for months.

Working with the mesoscopic[4] imaging of the monkey's inferior parietal lobule, Milena Raffi and I found a beautiful map of "navigational motion." Navigational motion is what you see as you move through the world. When you are moving down a ski slope, dodging past long drops, or cruising through a quiet stretch, your eyes are taking in an enormous volume of visual information. And if this information is allowed to get a bit simpler, it can become a visual stimulus that can be studied.

In our studies, a monkey would play a video game in which he had to fixate on a single red dot on a screen while a hundred white dots moved away from the fixation point. The appearance is like driving at night, with headlights through a blizzard. At some random time, the white dots would move randomly. The monkey would release a lever for a reward.

Testing different types of motions, we could assess their effects using close, detailed, eight-by-ten-millimeter pictures of the cortex. These mesoscopic pictures were measured from the reflected light shone onto the brain's surface. So if the representation of a rightward-moving stimulus was on, a particular motion would move across the cortex and lead to a particular type of reflected light. When the representation of a leftward-motion stimulus was on, the reflected light, the mesoscopic images, would be different.

Thus we could compute a colorful map, a functional architecture, of these different motions from the sensitive mesoscopic images we took of the brain. The bits of cortex that respond to the blizzard-driving scenario were purple; the bits that respond to the steering wheel spun clockwise were red, and so forth. At first, it was very satisfying to see the images form and build.

There was only one problem. When we repeated the experiment the next day, we found another nice colorful map of motion, but it did not align with the previous day's map. This situation, of course, frustrated us, as one of the hallmarks of good science is its reproducibility. Were we getting these patterns by doing something wrong or was something happening that was indicating a truth?

We found no fixed representation, at least for the inferior parietal lobule that we were studying. We asserted that the association cortex was generating new representations, new maps, all the time. As we honed our temporal analysis, we found these changes occurring in tens of seconds or less. The functional architectures, which we expected to be stable based on Hubel and Wiesel's seminal studies, kept changing under our mesoscope.

As we struggled to write up these frustrating results, other well-established principles and data seemed to get in the way. Many researchers had studied the inferior parietal lobule before us; all had used a single electrode, recording from a single neuron. They would study a neuron under a range of conditions and compute the averages of multiple tests. Some neurons would show statistical differences across these averages; others would not. Undeniably we had reported similar data—I published papers of this sort for more than twenty years.

When a single neuron is studied electrically, as I and others had done for years, the disorder is revealed in the variability that we, in our infinite wisdom, averaged away. This is ideal for finding out the nature of the representations of single cells, but misleading when considering the complexity of the true neural computation. It was the nature of the field and the questions we all asked that blinded us to the importance of the trial-by-trial variability. I could not make sense of the temporal variability and considered it to be "noise."

In the mesoscopic imaging experiments, however, we could observe an image of the primate brain in action; we could record from hundreds of thousands of sites (not neurons) at once. In a single trial, we could see across the cortex a *spatial* pattern of activity that was not simply "noise."

Putting these two results together was not conceptually easy. On one side was the edifice of studies from single neurons. All would acknowledge variability in the activity at a single recording site, with most of us excluding the changes over time from direct consideration. On the other side, our novel mesoscale maps changed from day to day, almost from moment to moment. Within each temporal mesoscale snapshot was a spatial order. The single-unit studies and the mesoscale-imaging results seemed to come from two separate brains. It did not compute.

The key to our finally understanding was accepting that functional architectures, the "advanced" maps of the brain, are dynamic and malleable. Each moment brings input from the outside world. The animal is selecting represented goals, assigning value to items in the world. The motivational state—be it hunger, thirst, craving for affection—has its representation in the brain. All these and more are being combined in different ways, putatively giving rise to our outward observed behavior, to consciousness.

We proposed that the brain finds a new solution every time its cognitive parts are challenged by input from many of its other parts. Particular cortical machinery answers particular types of questions, but each solution is scattered across the cortical surface. The recorded mesoscale patterns reflect constraints of the cortical machinery. Although it is almost impossible to keep every input identical, we had great control over the actual visual inputs, as well as the monkey's focus of attention and limb movements. But much more was happening in the monkey's brain. This constant selection of inputs through computation changed the maps.

We now believe that the functional architecture of the inferior parietal cortex is constantly modified in response to the changing internal and external world.

The advantage created by a scheme of cortical processing in which the neurons work in concert to find distributed solutions through variable spatial and temporal interaction is three-fold. First and foremost, in this scheme, no neuron in the thinking parts of the brain is dedicated to a highly specific representation. The computational machinery of the neural circuits can be reused as needed, which increases processing power and gives the cortex a great deal of flexibility for confronting diverse challenges.

Second, it allows processing to be efficiently carried out in the relatively small amount of cortical real estate dedicated to cognitive functions. In the visual system of a monkey, the area of the earliest primary visual cortex, VI, with a static and fixed mapping, is about the size of a credit card. This functional architecture represents at least four characteristics of the visual world: retinal location, orientation, left versus right eye, and color.

However, the inferior parietal lobule has neurons that represent many more characteristics: different eye positions in the orbit, the location of a visual stimulus in the world, spatial attention in many forms, navigational motion, hand position, eye movements, three-dimensionality from pairs of images, and reward. And the inferior parietal lobule does all of this in an area the size of half of the fingernail on your pinky finger.

If an intelligent brain maker wanted to spread out the processing of all cognitive spatial features with collections of neurons tied to particular features, it would take at least twice the area of early visual cortex. As we can easily define at least fifteen of these types of areas, that brain would be too large, too hot, and too heavy to have survived natural selection or passed through the birth canal.

Third, this scheme of cortical organization can support introspection. The cortical machinery can act solely on internal signals, unfettered by external events, collecting information from multiple cortices and passing them on to others. In one sense, the inferior parietal lobule really never has explicit knowledge of whether the arriving action potentials were triggered by a sensory event or some internal event, such as a thought. Its remoteness from pure sensory input makes it more prone to process intracerebral rather than sensory information, as Mountcastle noted from purely anatomical considerations in *The Mindful Brain*.[5] How the internal activity becomes a conscious thought is clearly a crucial and wide-open question, but these association areas are the ideal substrate to look for an answer or generally study mechanistically high cognition.

The type of static and fixed mapping that occurs in VI has historically been thought to underpin cortical processing. One reason for this conclusion is that in VI each nerve fiber consistently codes a labeled line, which represents a particularly inviolable piece of information. Such concepts stem from the early nineteenth century. Müller (1833) wrote of the "Law of Specific Nerve Energies"; Helmholtz (1867), of "labeled lines"; James (1890), of "loop lines." Donald Hebb relied on these ideas for his "resonating circuits." In Hubel and Wiesel's Ferrier Lecture (1971), the key to the concept of the functional architecture is the mapping of each visual feature on the cortex, making it accessible and organized for further processing. More recent studies expand this mapping idea into a plethora of visual cortical areas, each with a line carrying a set of visual characteristics.[6]

The most serious implication of the idea that the basis for cortical processing is a rapidly changing and adapting cortical area rather than a fixed cortical representation is that "labeled" lines do not simply lose their label, their identity; they do not survive at all.

If this is the case, cortices that need to interpret these unlabeled lines must do so using combinatorics of the preceding and following areas. For example, prefrontal cortical areas that receive inferior parietal lobule output must take spatial and temporally varying signals from multiple areas, combine them, and then realize a new representation, again distributed across a population. It is a new cortex, fraught with diversity, potent with possibility. From such diversity, from such potential can arise the fullness of experience of the entire brain. What is needed is a new way of thinking about cortical activity, of interacting areas working in concert to neurally select and sustain essential characteristics. The break from the machine-like view of cortex could be the link that allows a fully synthetic brain to join possibility and actuality to form thought and consciousness.

TEN

WAITING FOR THE TRAIN TO BALTIMORE

I am off to a train bound for Baltimore to visit Vernon Mountcastle. The core of the question I am taking to him is in a short sentence from the article that Milena Raffi and I published on attentional maps in the parietal cortex:

> It has not escaped our notice that the on-line neural construction of the patches would permit this portion of association cortex to subserve a multitude of cognitive processes, as a function of the ongoing inputs and behavioral state.[1]

As we saw in the last chapter, our study extended the idea, dating from the late 1800s, of a wiring diagram for cortical organization. Much of the modern study of the cortical underpinnings of vision is built on this core concept. Particular

locations or features in the world translate to particular locations in the cortex. In this way of thinking, it easily follows that
these features are laid out in an organized map across the surface
of the brain.

In the 1950s, Mountcastle and others found the first
evidence for a second level of organization, going perpendicular
to the cortical surface. They used a new technology (event
related potentials) that involved inserting fine microelectrode
wires into the brain that evaluated the activity of single neurons
as they altered the sensory inputs. The resulting "minicolumns"
had one modality represented; the initial findings were of columns of neurons with the same somatosensory signals from
surface touch and deep pressure. These columns were most
often dominated by the incoming signals; so that Müller's Law
of Specific Energies held. In other columns, however, intracortical processing—the interactions between neurons *within* an
area—dominated.

Kuffler, Hubel, and Wiesel initiated studies in the visual
cortex that were similar to Mountcastle's somatosensory measurements. They found that the structures in the primary visual
cortex were almost crystalline, so the work was fruitful. Gordon
Holmes had been the first to observe the structure for locating
the image on the eyeball—the retinotopic map. Kuffler, Hubel,
and Wiesel found columns for the orientation of a bar and for
the right and left eyes. Later studies even found small patches
for color embedded in these columns. There were columns all
the way down. Hubel and Wiesel coined the term "functional

architectures" for these replicating columns and structures. Others observed similar functional architectures in other parcels of the cortex. For example, motion area, MT, had a retinotopic map with motion and orientation embedded within it.[2]

This approach culminated with Felleman and Van Essen's overwhelming connectional diagram.[3] Each box had a map of some visual feature—motion, color, orientation, location—and these maps were also seen for the somatosensory and the auditory signals. This picture of cortex as a series of complex wiring diagrams between neurons has remained steadfast in our collective neuroscience consciousness. Neurons sent axons, little wires, labeled with information. There were wires for the color red, wires that transmitted motion, wires that said a face is present. Each type of wire—red, motion, face—was grouped with its own area. When any group connected to the next area, they were ordered, making the next step of processing relatively straightforward.

Although the concept of an organized map worked very well for the sensory and motor cortices (as in the homotypical cortex), it was not so clear for the "smarter" cortices. These were the areas in the middle—not necessarily sensory and not necessarily motor—called association cortices.

Mountcastle, recording from the heterotypical association parietal cortex in the behaving monkey, found a novel arrangement. Adjacent columns appeared to have different higher-order properties. He proposed a "salt-and-pepper" hypothesis for columns in the inferior parietal lobule. According to this theory, different sensory and motor modalities would organize in columns; these columns would intersperse across the cortical surface much as salt and pepper would intermix on a tablecloth near a sloppy diner's plate. Such an arrangement would nicely subserve interactions between somatosensory processes and vision, but understanding projections of connectivity to other cortical areas was not a natural consequence of Mountcastle's theory.

In an essential way, his salt-and-pepper view of association cortex violated the precept so widely supported by elegant studies of vision, where cortex consisted of a series of highly ordered and structured maps with subsequent hierarchical rules to extract more and more interesting "stuff." Neurons and areas for every aspect of visual experience (color, motion, faces) could all be constructed in this manner.

In this orderly view of the cortex, there was no apparent conceptual room for the disorderly salt-and-pepper micro-columns. How could such mixed projections be used in a system of orderly maps with nice wiring diagrams? How would neurons sort out the mixed-up signals from axons in a salt-and-pepper organization?

In our five-year attentional-map experiment, Milena Raffi and I trained the monkey to shift his attention right and left while he stared at a red dot on the computer screen. We used a highly sensitive camera to take pictures of the monkey's neural activity across the cortical surface.

One-millimeter colored patches of the cortex matched up with the monkey's right and left focus of attention. We were thrilled. The images nicely fit the dogma of a mapped wiring diagram of the brain. We had found the first trace of the monkey's thinking—of his attention—mapped across the cortical surface. Although other patchy maps of cortical columnar structure—the lattice-like structures of orientation, of color, of motion—had been published, no one else had ever seen a cognitive ability mapped across the cortex.

There was only one small problem, and it took us three years to solve it: The patch-like, columnar structure of attention changes over time.

Science relies on reproducibility. Each day we could get the map with spatial attention patches of the same size, but their location always shifted. We tried but failed to force consistent results—systematizing every step of the study. We failed. The monkey's brain insisted on being mutable.

This result was even worse than Mountcastle's salt and pepper heresy. Each day, someone was randomly stirring up the grains of salt and pepper. Our results were even worse for a wired view of the brain. The maps of attention were mixed in time, but not in space.

It took us a long time to discard our way of thinking about how a region of cortex works. If it was true that a single neuron could have different views of the world at any one time, a local-circuit, organizational principle would be variable in time. At some point, a gray pepper wire might carry a white salt signal.

Some researchers have argued for active changes in circuitry over time. Michael Merzenich described a somatosensory cortex that could be remapped after a drastic peripheral change, such as losing a finger. Ed Callaway, my summer colleague at Salk, speaks of circuits being turned on and off, brought into and out of play. Francis Crick wrote of neuronal ensembles being formed to match the moment. Gerald Edelman wants the brain to be a jungle of competing, evolving neural connections.

The trick is that not only will the local circuits need switching, but so will the intracortical circuits. When the parietal maps change, the readout areas will also have to change. It was hard to see how so many circuits could change so rapidly. It was hard to believe in a central control booth. Rodolfo Llinas proposes the thalamus as the controller. Edelman speaks of the cerebral appendages modulating these changes. Yet what could be in charge of such an overarching process?

After three years of considering the images we had collected, we published our findings. The monkey's brain had forced us to realize that the dogma would not hold for homotypical association cortex. In our short sentence, we argued for a new view of a very flexible cortex, one that could encode a diversity of opinion. Perhaps when we are free of the constraints of the Law of Specific Energies, we can have a model for brain that is permissive enough to allow the full range of diversity that occurs at every moment, with every thought.

Diversity. Is it like this in the brain? This freedom to be many substantiations of a flavor—or a sensation or a motor movement—separated in space and time, means that we can point at and understand the flexibility for real thoughts.

It became of the utmost importance to demonstrate this useful variability that coexists with spatial order. So many papers, even now, continue to average and ignore the trial-by-trial variability. The current rage is to analyze a special electrical signal, called local field potentials, to collect from many neurons at once, perform hefty computations, and compute "oblated spheroidal" or a fast Fourier transform. Yet for all our computational sophistication, in the end, everyone simplifies by adding up the parts and dividing by "N"—by averaging.

These are the ideas I want to sift through with Vernon Mountcastle.

My train is soon to depart. I need to go up to the platform.

———

The taxi deposits me at the Johns Hopkins University undergraduate campus. I am a bit early, but the paths are familiar to me, as the lay of the land is just as Google Earth led me to expect. I find the long round driveway. This is a campus with large expanses of grass, buildings of local red brick, trees not terribly old. A clock tower across the quad, and students roaming about. It is not inner-city Newark. I sit upstairs near the library, having found that the entrance to the stacks is blocked by a security station. To my left is the necessary espresso machine. To the right, the green sward. The coffee counter worker cracks the metal filter against the wood block, dumping the old grinds. Out around me, the blue sky is wrapped without a cloud.

I had known of Vernon Mountcastle from my earliest days as a graduate student. A postdoctoral fellow at McGill, Ian Hunter, was criticizing the Nobel Prize decision for 1981. He said the Nobel Committee was unfair to exclude Mountcastle from the prize in Medicine. Mountcastle, this erudite young scientist said, had discovered the cortical column, the mapping of the sense of touch across the cortex. "How much more had Hubel and Wiesel done?" Yet they shared that year's award for their discoveries on the functional architecture of visual cortex.[4]

My postdoctoral research settled on the inferior parietal lobule, the same cortical area that Mountcastle had tried his best to understand a decade earlier. Richard Andersen, my post-doctoral advisor, who had worked with Mountcastle, told of a disciplined scientist, assiduous in his desires to understand the enigmas of the association cortex. We began our work on this tough nut, using electrical measurements of brain activity while monkeys did complex visual tasks. We then correlated these measurements with the anatomical connections we obtained by looking at a thinly sliced and stained brain tissue.

During one annual Society for Neuroscience meeting, Carmen Cavada was presenting her recent findings on the connections of the inferior parietal lobule. It irked me, for Cavada and her advisor, Patricia Goldman-Rakic, had just renamed all the subdivisions of this area.

> What's in a name? that which we call a rose
> By any other name would smell as sweet.[5]

I should not have cared that Cavada and Goldman-Rakic had renamed 7ip, the lateral parietal area we named LIP, or that PO on the medial surface of the brain was now called 7m. But I was a young (and foolish) Turk, so in the questions following the presentation, I pointed out that these new names were superfluous and would only serve to confuse everyone else. I sat down feeling quite proud of myself.

To my right, one seat away, an older, well-dressed man leaned over and said, "You were exactly right. All these names are confusing matters." And then he reached and formally introduced himself. "I am Vernon Mountcastle."

Over the years, we got to know each other a bit better, mostly through chance meetings at conferences. I had invited myself to the Bard Laboratories at Johns Hopkins University to watch his monkeys in action. But we hadn't had the in-depth discussion I craved of the enigmatic inferior parietal cortex.

On this visit, Mountcastle asked me the conventional questions, family questions: where did I live, what was my neuroscience center like? Where I had studied? Who were my advisors?

He was surprised to find out that Richard Andersen was not my thesis advisor, but had supervised my postdoctoral work.

We moved on to talk about his newest accomplishment. He showed me the table of contents from his book that was being published that day.[6] He pulled out some manuscript pages on the connections of the prefrontal cortex, the seat of our richest brain experiences. "This might interest you." I skimmed through it.

"How does he do this?" I thought to myself. How does he get to write this all down?

I took a deep breath. I had to get to my problems with his cortices. First I had to explain the optical imaging showing that eye position was mapped across the cortical surface. This took a while, my hands fluttering as I tried to get my findings visualized.

Then I started to describe the representation of attention on the cortical surface, that Milena and I had seen attentional patches, and how they moved. I kept jumping ahead to the punch line. "No labeled lines."

I was trying to explain five years of work in as many minutes.

Mountcastle asked me how attention could, each day, move the representation on the cortex. I found it hard to hit the correct level of explanation. Even though we were both studying the same square centimeter of cortex, we lacked a common language.

I tried to explain that the dogma—that optically imaged architectures were based upon wiring—was irrelevant because we were looking at imaged structures that entirely represented function. I also explained that this led to a deeper and inescapable problem: How would an area interpret these signals?

My explanation was perhaps no more clear to him than that last paragraph was to you. Although the explanation came out all wrong, in jargon and in jerks, he did get my point about changing representations of attention on the cortical surface. This he got.

Mountcastle proposed that variation in impinging inputs caused the variation in the representations of the inferior parietal lobule. It was clear that he saw the organization of a cortical area as primarily reflecting the inputs. He saw the variability we had measured as a result of other cortical areas feeding in temporally varying information. The signals in the inferior parietal areas reflected the variation of the inputs.

He said that if we were right, we needed to show another associational area having equally variable representations. He pointed to the prefrontal-cortex chapter he had handed me. Would prefrontal cortex have equally variable representations?

Indeed, it should be possible to see a spatial correlation between the patches in the two areas. The inferior parietal and the prefrontal areas are interconnected; perhaps we could observe them changing together and the labeled connections shifting together. Would they still be labeled lines?

By the time we got to the point of giving up on labeled lines as a working system for sharing information, it was time for lunch.

As we walked over to the faculty dining room, he spoke of his Mind/Brain Institute. I could feel that Mountcastle was the holder of the flame, the ideals of the Institute. His colleague, Kenneth Johnson, had been the pragmatic chair. Johnson's death in May at age sixty-six had struck Mountcastle hard.

What was it Francis Crick said to me? "You know you are old when the ambassadors look young." Vernon kept speaking of Ken. Losing Ken was clearly to him like losing a son. At eighty-eight, many of your friends have died, and this was the case for Vernon Mountcastle. Max Cowan was gone. Patricia Goldman-Rakic gone. These people had died, leaving us with unfinished work.

As we walked from lunch, it was a most beautiful day. The weather was perfect, the sun out. Afterward, he sent me to visit some of his colleagues. By the time I came back, Mountcastle had sketched out some columns, with inputs arising at the left from pulvinar fed by cholinergic inputs. To the right, he had adrenergic inputs. I would have enjoyed discussing the role of diffuse connections leading to self-organization. But after three hours, it was time to go.

I didn't really get to explain my main research problem. And I didn't get the epiphany I sought. But Mountcastle did draw a set of columns—cholinergic and adrenergic inputs labeled. And after I told him about my studies, he had asked, "What would happen to the attention signal if you block adrenergic input?" He stressed the most important result was to confirm this in another area. We both thought that prefrontal was the most obvious candidate. How would this plan fly as a grant?

The visit was what it was. I had sought an epiphany. Vernon Mountcastle was still sharp, but as he said, "I am eighty-eight." At eighty-eight, science is still alluring and a true love; yet so is a wife and the end of a long, meaningful life.

ELEVEN

TRIUMVIRATE

Science is very slow. Some of my studies take months, some years, and some go on throughout life. Friendships casually formed become the basis of my lifework. There is mystery in this. I did not plan at sixteen; I did not write a set of specific aims. The science and I evolved organically.

Ehud Isacoff and I met in Montreal on a green field on Mont Royal off Avenue Parc with a simple Frisbee. I was eighteen; Ehud seventeen. I was studying physics; Ehud, biology. Our only thing we had in common was a heavily attended Biology 102 course taught by John Southin.

John pushed Lederberg, petri dishes, bacterial DNA, genes, and biological logic down our throats. His massive Biology 102 course was unlike the other introductory courses we attended.

He wrote his own textbook, which read more like Lewis Carroll's puzzles in logic than biology.[1] John induced us to read primary research publications, as well as to question hypothesis and evidence. His tutorial was not remedial; maybe twenty out of the three hundred Bio 102 students started it, but only a handful endured to the end.

John shone in teaching and the doing of science, and his apartment in the McConnell Hall Residence, where he was director, was unlike anything Ehud or I had seen before. It was walled with books ranging beyond our tyro scientific pursuits. There was an entire block of shelves containing poetry, another of prose, and another on human sexuality. He would hold forth in his handmade rocker, one leg folded under him, squeaking as he rocked. Behind him on his cinderblock wall were verses from Whitman's "Leaves of Grass." Little did we know, while throwing a Frisbee on the green dingle in Montreal, that John would become the first exemplar of the kind of life we wanted to live.

Ehud and I traveled in different circles for most of our undergraduate years. Ehud enjoyed molecular biology and continued in John's footsteps; his senior independent study was isolating histones from sea urchins. I finished my physics degree and entered the doctoral program in physiology to study biophysics, and sodium pumping in rabbit vagus nerves as a model of learning in synapses. Graduate students must teach, and so I selected the neurobiology laboratory course.

In Ronald Chase's neurobiology laboratory course, I instructed Ehud and the other students in various classic preparations.

We saw how the ganglia in the crayfish nerve cord controlled locomotion and how the giant American cockroach tail cerci triggered an escape response. To see real synaptic potentials, we placed tiny glass microelectrodes into giant neurons in the somatogastric ganglion of snails.

As the teaching assistant, I prepared the experiments. For the experiment that examined the junction between a frog's sciatic nerve and muscle, first you had to pith each frog. This consisted of placing it in ice water, and when this cold-blooded vertebrate stopped moving, inserting a needle into the base of its brain and swinging it around inside the skull to shred the brain. I would give the brain-dead frog to a pair of students and they would begin their experiment. The sciatic nerve in the thigh would be exposed, hopefully not split in half by the student's scalpel. Tiny silver hooks would be placed on the nerve and small electrical currents from a Grass stimulator passed through wire, hook, and nerve.

If everything was done right, the gastrocnemius muscle would twitch each time a button was pushed on the Grass. The students would alter the electrical stimulation and monitor the changes in strength of the muscle's pull. Finally they would cut the nerve out of the leg, place it in a Plexiglas box with ten silver wires as supports, and attach the Grass stimulator to one pair of wires. A second pair of wires, as distant as possible from the first, was connected to a recording oscilloscope—essentially a television display of the electrical actions in the nerve. The axons within the Grass box would initiate the action potential and the oscilloscope would record it.

The time between the stimulus and the recorded action potential demonstrated how fast information could travel in a nerve. It was like measuring the time in a race between the firing of the starter gun and the crossing of the finish line. Measurements from all of the animals studied in that class— including the cockroach, crayfish, and snail—formed a perfect survey of the state of neuroscience in 1980.

Ehud's and my first collaboration began the next semester. Ehud had treated twenty chickens with pesticide to examine its effects on the myelin in their brains. He performed biochemistry on the myelin, and I examined the conduction velocity of the nerve fibers in the sciatic nerves. The design was simple. We would sacrifice the chickens. Ehud would remove the brain from the head, and I would remove the sciatic nerve from the drumstick.

What happened was comical in a way. As we were two city boys, of course we had no idea how to kill a chicken. We spoke with other graduate students. One Iraqi student said that in his hometown, he would simply rapidly twirl the chicken over his head and snap its neck. Ehud and I could not fathom this. We spoke with the animal facility people and found that there was a small animal guillotine we could use. We were relieved. Simply put the chicken in the guillotine and step down on the pedal. We would need to hold the body in a drain until it stopped struggling, but that we could do.

One Saturday morning we arrived at McGill Medical School and set up all our equipment. Ehud was on the fourteenth floor making his solutions, and I set up all my electronics on the eleventh floor. We headed up to the sixteenth floor to sacrifice the animal. There was one problem. The guillotine was locked away. Being resourceful twenty-year-olds, we hit on a plan right away. I would cycle home and get my Chinese meat cleaver and sharpening stone.

We sat on the floor in the animal facility honing the knife. Ehud then held the body of the chicken and I pulled gently on the chicken's comb, stretching the neck out. I raised my right arm high. One two! One two! And through and through. The Chinese blade went snicker-snack!

Ehud held the chicken's body. Ehud was the one struggling with the spasms of the chicken, keeping it from running around the room, holding its severed neck in the drain. And I was the one staring at the chicken's head. It blinked at me. One two. One two. Its eyes opened and closed. Ehud and I were still. It was quiet. We did not laugh. We looked at each other. This was not easy to do.

We remembered with a jolt what we had to do. Ehud put the head in ice and rushed down to the fourteenth floor to dissect the brain and extract the myelin. I took a scalpel, reassuring instrument, and removed the two drumsticks and rushed down to the eleventh floor. I placed the leg on the dissecting tray, and with a scientific delicacy so distant from the moments on floor sixteen, I removed the sciatic nerve and placed it in the Plexiglas recording chamber appropriated from the undergraduate neurobiology laboratory. Chicken schmaltz floated in the chamber.

I stimulated the nerve and photographed the resulting compound action potentials, calculating the conduction velocity of the insecticide-treated and control chicken sciatic nerves.

One chicken was enough for us that day. Ehud and I cleaned up and headed home in the evening chill, somber.

The next weekend we made sure we had the guillotine available.

Our energy was youthful. We would elevator up to the animal facility on sixteen, guillotine the chicken, elevator back to our respective labs for our measurements. All weekend. In the end twenty chickens were studied.

When Ehud graduated, he put aside his beloved histones and molecular biology, and I recruited him to join me with Dick Birks for our synaptic studies of learning. There were countless nights of two young men, breaking from their recordings to eat black Russian bread from the Saint Laurent Bakery with cheese from the Patisserie Saint Denis. It is always the nights I remember, and the food. Certainly we must have discussed science, our results, their meaning, but that is not what memory recalls.

I finished my degree first, heading west to the Salk to work with Richard Andersen, going as far from the biophysics of the synaptic learning as possible, leaving Ehud to finish his degree with Dick Birks. I had thought Ehud had forgotten about his sea urchins and molecular biology. In all our late night meals, I had no inkling that he was planning a triumphant return to molecular biology.

Ehud headed to the University of California, San Francisco, and like me, also headed as far as possible from synaptic physiology. Ehud and Lily Jan were among the first experimentalists to manipulate the genetic sequence of ionic channels to understand their function.

In Pasadena, Ed Callaway studied nerves and muscles in graduate school, as I had studied vagus nerves. For both of us, it was a step to the brain.

In grad school, I studied very small-diameter nerve fibers in the vagus nerve of a rabbit.[2] Birks and I were not directly interested in the vagus nerve. We really wanted to know how the tiny boutons of nerve terminals released neurotransmitters in the nervous system. Birks had discovered that grouping nerve impulses in time into tightly compressed short groups (or bursts) would increase the amount of acetylcholine release. It was a mechanism for learning.

For his thesis, Ed studied synapse formation between nerves and muscles.[3] He also worked on rabbits, using a leg muscle as a model for the formation of synapses. In the soleus muscle, a unique relationship forms between nerves and muscle fibers as the animal develops. Each muscle fiber is excited by only one nerve. Ed and his thesis advisor, David Van Essen, used this neuromuscular junction to examine the rules governing the formation of the one-to-one relationship.

In his influential 1949 book, *The Organization of Behavior*, Donald O. Hebb suggested a particular rule for the strengthening of synapses, for learning. The synapse would be strengthened if activity occurred both presynaptically and postsynaptically. Multiple inputs could compete for a single postsynaptic target, with the input that fired most often in correspondence with the target winning out. This "Hebbian rule" underpinned most models of learning in those years.

Ed and David posited a competition among the nerve fibers, causing the increased use that would lead to the formation of more synapses. They tested this idea by shutting off some of the inputs to the nerve fibers. Unexpectedly, they found that decreased use, rather than increased use, formed more synapses—"a finding," they wrote, "opposite to that expected if the neuromuscular junction operated by classical 'Hebbian' rules of competition."[4]

Meanwhile, for my postdoctoral work, I had decided to study the "real" brain, in monkeys. I was fed up with a sliced up, stripped down model. I wanted the real thing.

I was occasionally lucky enough to attend the Helmholtz Club, and so met David Van Essen, one of the first of a new breed of monkey researchers to conduct computational explorations of the neurons in the brain. He invited me up to Caltech to see his laboratory, or more likely, I invited myself. He walked me around his laboratory; it was a warren of rooms, some for electrophysiological recordings of anesthetized monkeys, some for a new optical imaging setup, and still others for piles of computational equipment. In the back corner of a room that seemed far from all the other rooms, Ed Callaway was working on the rabbit neuromuscular junction.

I thought this was pretty neat. Even though I was running from biophysics, I knew that one day my science would encompass all the different levels. Van Essen showed me that it was possible to study synaptic transmission, and he did monkeys too! And I had just met Ed for the first time.

My time at the Salk was ending. I almost decided to join David Van Essen's laboratory for a second postdoctoral fellowship, but the lure of working with Nobel Laureate Torsten Wiesel at Rockefeller University in New York City was too great.

So I packed my things, and on April Fools' Day of 1987, I arrived at the Rockefeller University. The Rockefeller was not at all like the Salk. Out West, we were perched over the Pacific Ocean, a white ivory tower, the sun always shining, the view without limit. The Rockefeller sat on the East River of Manhattan, its buildings huge, impersonal. The sun was not always shining, and the view beyond the tidal strait of the East River was not infinite; it was of Roosevelt Island and Queens. The most profound difference for me was the loss of crosstalk between laboratories. At the Salk, lunch was outside looking toward the ocean. At the Rockefeller, the lunchroom was cavernous, seating hundreds.

The Rockefeller's saving grace was Torsten, his passion for the visual system, and his Laboratory for Neurobiology—five youngish investigators and a mix of postdoctoral trainees and graduate students.

There I met Ed Callaway again.

Ed and I had moved to Rockefeller to take on the cortex. He was there to build on his development studies with David Van Essen, which examined the importance of the visual environment in the creation of particular neuronal circuits. And he succeeded, doing intracellular work in monkeys and getting a job at the University of Colorado.

Ehud, Ed, and I were a perfect collaboration of three old and trusted friends, all experts in our domain, all charging forward to the same goal. My only concern was that I could keep up as these other two accelerated. We were trying to reach Francis Crick's dream: to understand consciousness, to peel back its dura, to seek inside the brain for the wet sloppy biological, neural, synaptic, and anatomical code that is our heritage and destiny.

None of us can do this alone. We can acquire our tools in part from others: in principle, molecular genetic constructs are available as soon as they are published, and optics and lasers can be bought. But what the three of us have is a unique interplay of ideas, approaches, and hypotheses.

Each summer, I take myriad lunchtime walks on the cliffs with Ed. Ehud and I have a rolling conversation of over thirty years. We cross paths, all three of us together rarely.

In essence, what we are doing is a simple plan, but a hard question. We are asking the cortex to tell us exactly what it does when it perceives, alludes, attends, plans, thinks. We have some hypotheses based on the giants whose shoulders we stand upon—part of our work is hypothesis-driven. But the bulk of it is an exploration, an exposure of the brain's actions. Our exploration is data-driven and reliant on the explosive range of techniques that Crick exhorted in the last twenty-five years of his life.

Here is one such experiment. In association cortices of the inferior parietal lobule, it seems that patches of cortical activity propagating across parietal topographies must arise from inter-actions, reentry, among neurons. Each patch is about one millimeter, the size of the Hubel and Wiesel hypercolumn, and should be constructed from a myriad of Mountcastle's micro-columns. Unlike in VI, where microcolumns tenaciously cling to their neighbors' function, something different is happening. Function is free to move from microcolumn to microcolumn, constantly reorganizing and seeking coalitions. Yet when we observe them mesoscopically, we see that order is somehow imposed on these patches of cortical activity. The most likely suspects are the axons that run horizontally with one-millimeter periodicities.

The long-range horizontal connections may, as Edelman's Neural Darwinism predicts, permit computations between microcolumns to form. These computations occur not in isola-tion, but through what Edelman calls reentry and others call feedback.[5] These roughly ten million neurons interact and com-pete with dozens of special cell types and equally as many neurotransmitters. It is an insanely wild choreography.

In our mesoscopic images, all of this detail is hidden. We see only the ebb and flow of thousands of dancers, each one lost to sight. When we try to watch individuals, stabbing at them with our sharp platinum-iridium electrodes, we glimpse tiny fractions of the dance, just one dancer, moving in position. We can see the patches only from afar; up close, they look like noise with just enough order for us to publish—poor approximations of the truth.

Enter molecular biology. Ed is deep in the midst of creating the means to isolate different neuronal types based on their genetic constituents and connectional strategies. Crick had laid the design specifications for three such tools in his 1979 *Scientific American* essay, "Thinking About the Brain."[6] The first tool should find every neuron connected to just one cell.[7] It took almost thirty years for this tool to be developed. Ian Wickersham, a remarkable graduate student, and Ed used the rabies virus. They broke the virus into two independent genetic parts to effect standard propositional logic onto anatomy. Neuron B would express a select genetic marker only if Neuron A had the protein coat of rabies *and* Neuron B had the core of rabies *and* the two neurons touched at a synapse. The development of this static anatomical marker of connectivity relies entirely on the addition of molecular biology to the systems neuroscience toolkit.

This tool allows us to delimit the anatomically defined cell assembly. At the very least, these cells touch each target through a synapse. Presumably these cells would be the primal element of cortical competition, related in part to Mountcastle's microcolumns and in part to the connectivity running between the columns.[8]

The simplest interpretation of these groups of neurons is that the rabies operationally defines an element of Hebb's cell assembly. These cells work together to construct visual representations. For example, in VI, the properties of a target neuron are defined by all of its inputs. The connectivity defines the function, so that if we understand the transmitters and the details well enough, we ought to be able to predict the response of the target cell. These operationally defined cell assemblies act conceptually much like Mountcastle's original idea of the microcolumn, which allows us to imagine a reductionist view of VI, where each element is understood. Voilà, we understand how VI works.

Whether this is correct for VI remains to be seen, but there must be some problems, a priori, in applying such concepts to the attentional patches in the inferior parietal lobule. When the patches are moving around on the cortical surface, elements of these anatomically defined cell assemblies do not always seem to be doing the same thing. It seems that at some moments, these cell assemblies could join up with a certain set of groups, and at others, with a different set of groups. The binding together would depend on the need and circumstance. Function overrides anatomy.

This is all very nice, but it is almost philosophy: words, hypothesis—without proof. One could almost reason it differently.

There could be groups of cells that are active together because they are anatomically bound. At times these groups of cells are tuned for one behavior; at other times, for another.

What if we think of the rabies-defined patches of neurons, the set of cells that is attached to one cell, as a basic neural assembly? It seems to me that if everything is anatomically based, this type of configuration forms the cell assembly. If function overrides anatomy (as in area 7a), these groups of cells could join up with other different groups depending on need and circumstance.

Such different neural strategies cannot be measured electrophysiologically because the direct anatomical connections between neurons cannot be assessed electrically. The only way to directly and simultaneously ask questions about the connectivity and the function is to use light in concert with molecular biology. This is where Ehud comes in. He specializes in genetically encoding light-emitting probes of neuronal activity. All those ionic channels that he had carefully sequenced and meticulously dissected can be used to measure neural activity.

So the next step, to examine the neural circuits underlying the moving attentional patches, can be taken by adding the genes for Ehud's probes into the rabies viruses. Doing this makes it possible not only to find connected cells, but also to watch their activity. Now we can label all of the connected cells and watch their activity using light. We can see what Hebb calls the neuronal assembly, what Koch and Crick call neural coalitions, and what Edelman calls selected neuronal groups.

The propagating attentional patches need to be observed at the microscopic level while the behaving monkey plays his attentional games. A final tool is needed—the ability to observe the actual neurons in the brain during behavior. Fortunately this ability was developed in the mid-1990s by remarkable neurobiologists and physicists: The two-photon scanning microscope, a laser microscope that uses nonlinear optics to penetrate up to half a millimeter into the cortex and resolve neurons and their structures at the submicron scale.[9] This microscope has altered how cells are observed in biological domains as diverse as the cell cycle and nematodes' molecular mechanisms of learning and memory. Most of the neuroscience was performed with this microscope under highly physically controlled conditions in anesthetized rats and mice or in a slice of brain tissue in a dish.

For Ed, Ehud, and me, the two-photon microscope is the one tool needed to observe these neuronal assemblies in the behaving monkey's brain. Over a period of three years, Barbara Heider and I adapted this microscope to the behaving monkey.[10] In our first test case in the primary visual cortex, we could see neurons that were genetically transformed and could assess their functional properties.

Our microscopic measurements are crude at this point. The quality of the images and the strength of the signals are not perfect. They are reminiscent of the initial electrical recordings of the early to mid-twentieth century: large tube amplifiers, the oscilloscopes to monitor the electrical signals of the cells, needed constant calibration. The resulting images were crude. Now electrical measurements of the brain's operations are crisp and clear.

We hope for similar developments over time, with the two-photon images of the genetically transformed neurons in the behaving monkey giving us sharp images of the entire neurons, their activity at each point nicely defined.

"To ask the hard question is simple," as the poet W. H. Auden observed.[11]

The hard question for us can now be exposed to the light. Do neurons that anatomically connect to a single cell remain part of the same coalition over time?

The experiment is easy enough to outline. Ed's propositional logic rabies virus is engineered to express Ehud's fluorescence sensor of activity. I put the viruses into the parietal cortex. The two-photon microscope assesses the activity of the neurons while the monkey performs the attentional task. What would the outcome be?

It could be that the brain would tell us the answer to the hard question. One outcome could be that when the monkey shifted his attention to one location, all the cells would light up and blink together. When the monkey's attention was shifted to a new location, they would cease to fire as a group. The selection group (or coalition) of cells would change its dependence on where the attention was placed. Such a result would speak to a remarkable role that physical connectivity between neurons would play in binding the neural elements together.

The alternative outcome is equally scintillating. Neurons would fire independent of the connectivity that was revealed by the rabies. Some of the interconnected neurons would fire when the monkey attended right, and others would fire when he attended left. That result would push function and competition to the forefront of how neurons interact to solve a cognitive problem in the association cortex.

Ed, whose laboratory is engrossed in the neural correlates of early vision, thinks that these flexible properties of association cortex are underestimated in early visual cortex. The small number of studies challenging early visual cortex with rich real-work stimuli are almost Precambrian. I hope that Ed will race forward and show that the circuits of early visual cortex are equally as "smart" as my parietal areas. Ed's studies have the advantage of a body of detail of neural circuits to build upon—much is his, and much belongs to the heritage accumulated since Hubel and Wiesel started in 1958. In time, he will want to wake up his monkeys, and I will be there to start his behaving studies, just as he has been there for me to start these virus studies in parietal cortex.

Ehud's drive for new sensors, for new ways to use light and molecular biology, will illuminate for us cortical types in ways still undreamed of. It may be a light sensitivity, a new cortical way for proteins to interact, or perhaps just a very sensitive potentiometer.

The interlocking of friendship and science augurs well, if not just for the science, for the completeness of our lives, our all too limited time as scientists.

TWELVE

CONSCIOUSNESS

I arrived at Oliver Sacks' home just after Jonathan Miller, who was devouring the sturgeon. "Like butter," I said, and helped myself to some brown bread and fish. Jonathan, a childhood friend of Oliver's whose many endeavors included directing opera, was talking about whether consciousness was amenable to scientific measurement. His argument was not one of a covert spiritualist—he argued that consciousness is unlike anything we have scientifically examined.

What does he mean? True, the brain is very, very complicated. True, almost no one can agree on a definition. True, everyone knows what their own consciousness is. But is its complexity unfathomable?

Consciousness arises from and is identical to the stuff of the brain. Can we get a scan of it? Only when our analysis and theory are broad enough to encompass consciousness, and to demonstrate the fine details of consciousness, will we have what is needed.

Jonathan asks, "Can science explain *art*?" Is art unlike anything we have scientifically studied? Some very good scientists try to see art through science's visual system, but Jonathan, Oliver, and I agree that their attempts at explaining art are bound to fail. Their theory of art is not nearly as well developed as their theory of brain.

Indeed, these scientists may not have the right sort of brain (or the right training) to understand art. We are (by definition) experts in our own disciplines. After all, how often does a true polymath come on the scene? After all this specialization, who can afford to be a polymath? How could science explain T. S. Eliot's[1]

> April is the cruelest month, breeding
> Lilacs out of the dead land, mixing
> Memory and desire, stirring
> Dull roots with spring rain.

Perhaps Jonathan's comment that consciousness is unlike anything science has studied is not quite right. Each field is a closed society with its own set of rules, eternally (one hopes) self-consistent. As each field matures, it spreads, at times questioning its own provenance.

Neuroscience is at a funny place. The wealth of details and understanding is exponential in its growth. For some neuroscientists, the goal is understanding neurological disease with its emphasis on molecular and cellular mechanisms. For me and many of my friends, the goal is to know the mechanisms for mind and brain. Consciousness is no different to us than a very complex neuronal circuit, emerging from interactions across multiple levels of explanation (as Marr nicely posited in 1982). We want to know consciousness, yet we discern the difference between understanding consciousness and its mechanisms and having insight into the first lines of Eliot's poem, *The Waste Land.*

The individuality of each of us is recognized by some scientists.[2] Yet can science measure the event of consciousness? Correlates have been and will continue to be found between neural activity and consciousness. But science may be able to say how each person will respond to Jonathan's operas only if scientists can incorporate the entirety of an individual's knowledge. And perhaps that is where scientists ought to draw the line. That individual's entirety of knowledge is that individual. It cannot be measured in a short brain scan or read out from all the trillions of synapses. That form of consciousness, the individual's consciousness, is not only in the realm of neuroscience; it is part of the complete landscape of knowledge. And that might just be something beyond the reach of science.

NOTES

Dedication

Bowl illustration by Jasmine J. A. Siegel; sunflower illustration by Zoe Julia Siegel.

Epigraph

Auden, W. H. "The Question." Copyright © 1933 by W. H. Auden. Reprinted by permission of Curtis Brown, Ltd.

Preface

1 Kandel, Eric R. 1976. *Cellular Basis of Behavior*. San Francisco: W. H. Freeman.

2 Kuffler, Stephen W., and John G. Nicholls. 1976. *From Neuron to Brain*, preface to first edition. Sunderland, MA: Sinauer Associates.

Chapter 1: *A Day in the Monkey's Brain*

1 This was made more than academically clear by my father's cerebellar stroke. He would tell me his mind remained clear, his thoughts strong, but he just could not communicate through his slurred speech. He still knew how to perform the most intricate dental procedures, but his hand could not, would not, listen.

2 Mathematics is the language of complete understanding. If the data can be captured by a mathematical model that predicts all past, present and future behavior, we "know" the underlying processes.

3 Marr, David. 1982. *Vision: A Computational Investigation into the Human Representation and Processing of Visual Information.* New York: W. H. Freeman.

Chapter 4: *Chaos Through the Looking Glass*

1 Edelman, Gerald M. 2004. *Wider Than the Sky: The Phenomenal Gift of Consciousness.* New Haven: Yale University Press, p. 35.

2 Glass, L. 1969. Moiré effect from random dots. *Nature* 223(5206): 578–580.

3 In this, Marr revealed a hope to achieve the same understanding of brain function that Watson and Crick had achieved for life in their model of DNA. He used the term "codon" to describe the attributes that would best activate a neuron. The selection of this word could be no accident; it was coined by Crick for a sequence of three nucleotides that define each amino acid.

4 Stent, Gunther S. 1972. Prematurity and uniqueness in scientific discovery. *Scientific American* 227(6): 84–93, 128.

5 Rockland, Kathleen S., and Jennifer S. Lund. 1982. Widespread periodic intrinsic connections in the tree shrew visual cortex. *Science* 215(4539): 1532–1534. Rockland and Lund write:

> How literally should we take the image of a cortical column
> as a functional entity, designed to segregate out different

submodalities? We might rather entertain the view of multiple repetitive structures intrinsic to the cortex, which may be adapted to fulfill a variety of functions. It may be useful to consider the vertical radial component of the cortex as enmeshed in an elaborate horizontal laminar organization, possibly in a multiple lattice-like design. Although the influence of each lattice could be translated through the cortical depth, this concept stresses the primacy of a particular lamina in elaborating a given function and underlines the importance of dynamic interconnections throughout the horizontal as well as the vertical extent of the cortex.

6 Squire, Larry R., ed. 2001. *The History of Neuroscience in Autobiography*, vol. 3, San Diego: Academic Press, p. 312.

7 Parent, P., and S. W. Zucker. 1989. Trace inference, curvature consistency, and curve detection. *IEEE Trans. Pattern Analysis and Machine Intelligence* 11(8): 823–839.

8 Zucker, S. W., and S. Davis. 1988. Points and endpoints: a size/spacing constraint for dot grouping. *Perception* 17(2): 229–247 (submitted 1985).

9 Carpenter, G. A., and S. Grossberg. 2003. Adaptive resonance theory, in Michael A. Arbib, ed., *The Handbook of Brain Theory and Neural Networks*, second ed. (pp. 87–90). Cambridge: MIT Press.

Chapter 5: Bright Moments

1 Barlow, H. B. 1972. Single units and sensation: A neuron doctrine for perceptual psychology? *Perception* 1(4): 371–394.

2 Talbot, W. H., I. Darian-Smith, H. H. Kornhuber, and V. B. Mountcastle. 1968. The sense of flutter-vibration: comparison of the human capacity with response patterns of mechanoreceptive afferents from the monkey hand. *Journal of Neurophysiology* 31(2): 301–334.

3 Fig. 25 of Mountcastle, V. B., R. H. LaMotte, and G. Carli. 1972. Detection thresholds for stimuli in humans and monkeys: comparison with threshold events in mechanoreceptive afferent nerve fibers innervating the monkey hand. *Journal of Neurophysiology* 35: 122–136.

4 Newsome, W. T., K. H. Britten, and J. A. Movshon. 1989. Neuronal correlates of a perceptual decision. *Nature* 341(6237): 52–54.

Chapter 6: *Eighth Avenue Line at Fourteenth Street*

1 Sacks, Oliver. 2004. Speed, *The New Yorker*, August 23: 60–69.

2 Actually, in 1984, you went to a teletype, dialed up with a modem to the Medline database, and used an awkward search syntax. You ended up with a long, continuous, faint dot-matrix printout.

3 Wilson, D. A. 1984. A comparison of the postnatal development of post-activation potentiation in the neocortex and dentate gyrus of the rat. *Developmental Brain Research* 16(1): 61–68; and Voronin, L. L., A. V. Bashkis, S. L. Buldakova, and V. G. Skrebitskiĭ. 1984. [Prolonged potentiation of responses of the neocortex of the intact brain and in vitro cortical slices]. *Fiziol Zh SSSR Im I M Sechenova* 70(8): 1167–77.

4 Shymko, R. M., and L. Glass. 1975. Negative images in stroboscopy. *Optical Engineering* 14: 506–507; Glass, L., and E. Switkes. 1976. Pattern recognition in humans: correlations which cannot be perceived. *Perception* 5(1): 67–72.

5 Schrauf, M., B. Lingelbach, and E. R. Wist. 1997. The scintillating grid illusion. *Vision Research* 37: 103–38.

6 Sacks, Oliver, and R. M. Siegel. 1990. Migraine aura and hallucinatory constants, in Sacks, Oliver, *Migraine*, rev. ed. New York: Vintage Books.

Chapter 7: *Modern Times*

1 One of my colleagues at Rutgers, Howard Poizner, has pointed out that this transformation was indeed one of great complexity due to the

invariance problem of speech. The same sequence of letters can give rise to two very different speech waveforms, depending on context. Almost any word will do. Take the word "about." The sound that we perceive as /b/ is very different when /b/ is in this phonetic context than when it is in another phonetic context, such as in "baby." The classic article on this issue is Liberman, A. M., F. S. Cooper, D. P. Shankweiler, and M. Studdert-Kennedy. 1967. Perception of the speech code. *Psychological Review* 74(6): 431–461. So indeed this was genuinely a hard problem, which still gives rise to controversies today.

2 Bliss, T. V. P., and T. Lømo. 1973. Long-lasting potentiation of synaptic transmission in the dentate area of the anaesthetized rabbit following stimulation of the perforant path. *Journal of Physiology* 232: 331–356.

3 Tsodyks, M. V., and T. J. Sejnowski. 1995. Rapid state switching in balanced cortical network models. *Network* 6(2): 111–124.

4 van Vreeswijk, C., and H. Sompolinsky. 1996. Chaos in neuronal networks with balanced excitatory and inhibitory activity. *Science* 274(5293): 1724–1726.

Chapter 8: *Visual Irredentism*

1 Malsburg, Christoph von der. 1981. The Correlation Theory of Brain Function, Internal Report 81–2, Max-Planck-Institut für Biophysikalische Chemie. Reprinted in E. Domany, J. L. van Hemmen, and K. Schulten, eds., 1994. *Models of Neural Networks II* (pp. 95–119), Berlin: Springer.

2 Gray, C. M., and Wolf Singer. 1989. Stimulus-specific neuronal oscillations in orientation columns of cat visual cortex. *Proceedings of the National Academy of Sciences USA* 86(5): 1698–1702. At one time, getting these preprints was easy. Now, the intense competition in science means you wait until the work is published before getting more than a taste.

3 I wrote to Malsburg about whether he had coined the term; he said that the word "bind" was used once by him.

4 Edelman, Gerald M., and Vernon B. Mountcastle. 1978. *The Mindful Brain: Cortical Organization and the Group-Selective Theory of Higher Brain Function*. Cambridge: MIT Press.

5 A recent theoretical model implements a reentry model to solve the segregation of foreground and background (Craft, E., H. Schütze, E. Niebur and R. von der Heydt. 2007. A Neural Model of Figure–Ground Organization. *Journal of Neurophysiology* 97(6): 4310–4326.

6 Edelman expanded on these ideas in his 1990 book *The Remembered Present: A Biological Theory of Consciousness* (New York: Basic Books) and later books.

Chapter 9: *Critique of Pure Cortical Topography*

1 Holmes, Gordon. 1945. Ferrier Lecture: The organization of the visual cortex in man. *Proceedings of the Royal Society of London, Series B, Biological Sciences*. 132(869): 348–361.

2 Hubel, David H., and Torsten Wiesel. 1977. Ferrier Lecture: Functional architecture of macaque monkey visual cortex. *Proceedings of the Royal Society of London—Series B: Biological Sciences* 198: 1–59.

3 There is an extensive literature on the effect of "severe perturbations" remapping the cortex, for example: Recanzone, G. H., M. M. Merzenich, W. M. Jenkins, K. A. Grajski, and H. R. Dinse. 1992. Topographic reorganization of the hand representation in cortical area 3b owl monkeys trained in a frequency-discrimination task. *Journal of Neurophysiology* 67(5): 1031–1056.

4 Imaging at the 0.01 to 1 millimeter scale allows us to see the brain's picture.

5 Edelman, G. M., and V. B. Mountcastle, eds. 1978. *The Mindful Brain: Cortical Organization and the Group Selective Theory of Higher Brain Functions*. Cambridge: MIT Press.

6 Felleman, D. J., and D. C. Van Essen. 1991. Distributed hierarchical processing in the primate cerebral cortex. *Cerebral Cortex* 1: 1–47.

Chapter 10: *Waiting for the Train to Baltimore*

1 Raffi, M., and R. M. Siegel. 2005. Functional architecture of spatial attention in the parietal cortex of behaving monkey. *Journal of Neuroscience* 25(21): 5171–5186. Our sentence was modeled after a similar one in Watson and Crick's 1953 paper: "It has not escaped our notice that the specific pairing we have postulated immediately suggests a possible copying mechanism for the genetic material." Its use reflected our admiration of the original study, the (perhaps misplaced) importance we attached to our own work, and, as we were writing soon after Crick's death, a wistful sigh at the end of an era.

2 Gattass, R., and Gross, C. G. 1981. Visual topography of striate projection zone (MT) in posterior superior temporal sulcus of the macaque. *Journal of Neurophysiology* 46(3): 621–638; Albright, T. D., R. Desimone, and C. G. Cross. 1984. Columnar organization of directionally selective cells in visual area MT of the macaque. *Journal of Neurophysiology* 51(1): 16–31.

3 Felleman, D. J., and D. C. Van Essen. 1991. Distributed hierarchical processing in the primate cerebral cortex. *Cerebral Cortex* 1: 1–47.

4 Roger Sperry also shared the award that year for his work on split-brain patients and elements of consciousness.

5 William Shakespeare, "Romeo and Juliet," Act 1, scene I.

6 Mountcastle, Vernon B. 2005. *The Sensory Hand: Neural Mechanisms of Somatic Sensation*. Cambridge: Harvard University Press.

Chapter 11: *Triumvirate*

1 Southin, John L. 1984. Inquiry and exploration in introductory science. *New Directions for Teaching and Learning* 20: 99–108.

2 Siegel, R. M., and R. I. Birks. 1988. A slow potassium conductance after action potential bursts in rabbit vagal C fibers. *American Journal of Physiology* 254: R443–R452.

3 Callaway, E. M., J. M. Soha, and D. C. Van Essen. 1987. Competition favouring inactive over active motor neurons during synapse elimination. *Nature* 328(6129): 422–426.

4 Callaway, E. M., J. M. Soha, and D. C. Van Essen. 1987. Competition favouring inactive over active motor neurons during synapse elimination. *Nature* 328(6129): 422–426.

5 The difference between the two is clearly made in Edelman's 1989 book, *The Remembered Present* (New York: Basic Books). Not only does reentry occur between micro-columns, but also between areas.

6 Crick, Francis. 1979. Thinking about the brain. *Scientific American* 241(3): 219–232.

7 There are two other tools: the ability to shut off specific neurons and the ability to differentially label visual areas. See Siegel, R. M., and E. M. Callaway. 2004. Francis Crick's legacy for neuroscience: between the α and the Ω. *PLoS Biology* 2(12): e419E. Ed is well underway for the second of Crick's tools—a way to shut off just one of the twenty neuronal cell types. When Francis first mentioned this to me sitting at a table at the westmost end of the Salk. I thought we would use killer antibodies. I was naïve.

8 All would seem perfect to explore the neural assemblies in monkeys. But there is one small difficulty. Neurons that have rabies die in short order; the rabies virus is too efficient in taking over the cell's protein synthesis machinery. The virus generates apoptotic proteins and massive amounts of the green jellyfish protein that soon kill the cell. This is not the best thing for chronic studies in trained primates. But someday. . . .

9 Denk, W., K. R. Delaney, A. Gelperin, D. Kleinfeld, B. Strowbridge, D. W. Tank, and R. Yuste. 1994. Anatomical and functional imaging of neurons using 2-photon laser scanning microscopy. *Journal of Neuroscience Methods* 54(2): 151–162.

10 This time overlapped with the same three years that Milena Raffi and I were convincing ourselves that attentional patches could indeed move.

11 Auden, W. H. "The Question." Copyright © 1933 by W. H. Auden. Reprinted by permission of Curtis Brown, Ltd.

Chapter 12: Consciousness

1 Eliot, T.S. "The Burial of the Dead," in *The Waste Land*. Used by permission of Faber and Faber Ltd.

2 Siegel, R. M. 1993. Seat of the will: a review of *Bright Air, Brilliant Fire: on the Matter of Mind* by Gerald Edelman, *BioScience* 43: 712–715.

Ralph Mitchell Siegel received his undergraduate and doctoral degrees at McGill University, and began his career as a research associate with Nobel Laureate Torsten Wiesel at Rockefeller University. He served as Visiting Scientist at IBM's Thomas J. Watson Research Laboratories before moving to Rutgers University, where he was Director of the Center for Computational Neuroscience and a Professor at the Center for Molecular and Behavioral Neuroscience. He was an Affiliated Research Fellow at the Neurosciences Institute in La Jolla, as well as a Visiting Sloan Center Scholar and a Crick-Jacobs Fellow at the Salk Institute for Biological Studies, until his death in 2011 at the age of 52.

Siegel began his career in the 1980s, just when the neuro-physiology of vision was coming into focus with the advent of new computing and imaging technologies. As a pioneer in the technique of mesoscopic imaging, he worked with some of the giants in vision science—Torsten Wiesel, Francis Crick, Tom Albright and others—and collaborated on a number of cases with the neurologist Oliver Sacks.

Siegel's work on parietal lobe neurons and the influence of eye position and attention on perception received many honors, including a National Science Foundation Career Award. He was a member of the AAAS, the Society for Neuroscience, the New York Academy of Science, the Biophysical Society, and the American Physiological Society. From 2006–2011, he served on the editorial board of *Brain Structure and Function*.

Tom Albright, a longtime friend and colleague at the Salk Institute, recalls, "From the earliest days of his scientific career, Ralph was an iconoclast—ever thinking outside the box, coura-geously questioning the perceived wisdom and pushing the boundaries of his field. At the same time, Ralph became known and loved far and wide for his extraordinarily passionate approach to science, family and friendship, his hearty *joie de vivre* and his generous spirit. Ralph thrived on his ability to excite, to provoke and to inspire those around him. He danced without pause through his short life."

INDEX